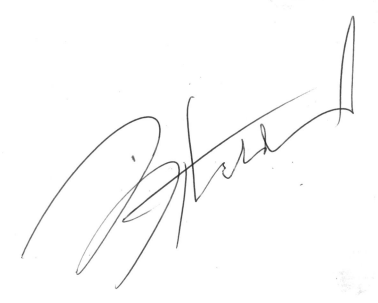

TERRY HITCHCOCK AND PETER JESSEN

A FATHER'S ODYSSEY

75 MARATHONS IN 75 DAYS

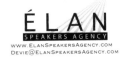

ÉLAN
SPEAKERS AGENCY
WWW.ElanSpeakersAgency.com
Devie@ElanSpeakersAgency.com

TERRY HITCHCOCK AND PETER JESSEN

A FATHER'S ODYSSEY

75 MARATHONS IN 75 DAYS

WITH JEFF TURNER AND KYLE GEARHART

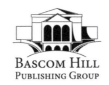

BASCOM HILL
PUBLISHING GROUP

Bascom Hill Publishing Group
212 3rd Avenue North, Suite 290
Minneapolis, MN 55401
612.455.2293
www.bascomhillpublishing.com

ISBN - 1-935098-13-6
ISBN - 978-1-935098-13-3
LCCN - 2008936348

Book sales for North America and international:
Itasca Books, 3501 Highway 100 South, Suite 220
Minneapolis, MN 55416
Phone: 952.345.4488 (toll free 1.800.901.3480)
Fax: 952.920.0541; email to orders@itascabooks.com

Cover Design by James Wilkinson
Typeset by Peggy LeTrent

Printed in the United States of America

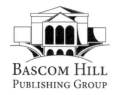

BASCOM HILL
PUBLISHING GROUP

TABLE OF CONTENTS

"Children are our future. Whether we are champions or challengers as we go through life, we need to continue to set examples for others to follow. When Terry and Chris set off to accomplish their impossible trek, it wasn't impossible to them. It was their dream and they knew they could be successful. As in any accomplishment, whether in the boxing ring or elsewhere, it takes training and hard work, being dedicated to your dream, and having a game plan. Terry and Chris are my heroes. They are everyone's heroes."

—*Scott LeDoux, a heavyweight fighter in the 1970's and early 80's. "The Fighting Frenchman", as he was known, twice fought for the World Championship.*

"There are many clichés about overcoming life's obstacles, such as turning your lemons into lemonade and every obstacle is God's opportunity. And they are all true. Yet, the greatest voice is the life that gives witness to these great truths – it is walking, or should I say running, in Terry's case, the talk, instead of simply talking the talk. Terry's life is an example that inspires all who encounter him."

—*Donna Rice Hughes, an Internet safety author, speaker and advocate. President of Enough Is Enough.*

"Terry's trek was a feat of feet, an unbelievable story of courage and dedication. Terry, with his son Chris, gave to all of us the focus and reason for our own lives. We all need to look around us and see if we too can find our own marathons to run. Terry and Chris believed in their dreams. We all need to do the same. Terry accomplished the impossible, but nothing is really impossible if we believe in ourselves. Terry's story is one of a real life Forrest Gump."

—*Tim VandeSteeg, CEO of Indiewood Pictures, a producer and director.*

"Life is precious and time is a key element. Let's make every moment count and help those who have a greater need than our own. Every day, we each have our own marathons to run. We train. We practice. We ask others for help and support … but we still have to run our own marathons. Terry showed us all how to run, to train and prepare, to believe, to live our lives and to make a difference in the lives of others. We can all help others. We just have to take that first step."

—*Harmon Killebrew, a member of the National Baseball Hall of Fame, 13-time All-Star, and Most Valuable Player in 1969, ending his career with 573 home runs.*

"Terry's ability to do what was deemed impossible is remarkable beyond words. His inspiration should change the thinking of those who haven't lived the life of a single parent or a child of want. Terry overcame all obstacles and told his story. He challenged the medical community to believe in him and not to say it couldn't be done ... Terry dreamed so that all children could dream."
—*Rob Gillio, M.D., a health care inventor and educator, and a passionate volunteer.*

"The future of our great country is predicated on the health and success of our children. They are our future. What Terry and Chris accomplished is an example of what we all need to strive for - to reach beyond, to believe in our dreams, and to work hard to make a difference in the lives of others. We too need to run our own daily marathons and to stand up and be counted."
—*U.S. Sen. Norm Coleman, of Minnesota, and former mayor of Saint Paul.*

"Winning a marathon has become synonymous with endurance and commitment. Imagine then what it must be like to run not one, but 75 consecutive marathons in 75 days. It has been done but once. The runner's name is Dr. Terry Hitchcock. His 1996 run from Minneapolis to Atlanta was an amazing demonstration of dedication and endurance. He too has a victory message. His is a message of how courage and commitment can overcome adversity. It is a story that every runner, every child, every family should read as they encounter boulders in their path or sand in their shoes on life's road to success."
—*Richard G. Marklund, Chairman of Phoenix New Castle Holdings Inc. and former Chairman of the Children Are Forever Foundation.*

"Terry's belief in his dream is an inspiration to all of those who have a task that seems unconquerable. The journey begins and you pick up speed and energy from others who also believe and dream. Together we can build the world that we believe in. Often it just takes the courage to begin, the courage to start. The commitment to follow comes from the collective strength of the wonderful people who come into our lives as a result of that first step."
—*Patty Wetterling, with her husband, in 1990 founded the Jacob Wetterling Foundation, four months after their son Jacob was kidnapped.*

"The world needs stories of triumph, passion and believing in oneself. The story of Terry Hitchcock and his son Chris is such a story. Children and families need to know that dreams do come true and that heroes can be anyone – including you."
—*Donna Smith, President and CEO of Cinema Completions International, and the first woman to head physical production at Universal Pictures.*

"We are all challenged to make a difference with our life. We are responsible for our effort, not the outcome. If we put 100 percent into the effort, the outcome will be good."
—*Mary Jo Copeland, founded Sharing and Caring Hands in 1985.*

"The dictionary defines perseverance as "adherence to a course of action, belief, or purpose". This is the embodiment of Terry. All the better that Terry is using his talents to help our children"
—*Martin J. Kanter, founder of Schechter Dokken Kanter, C.P.A.s and consultant.*

"Heroes guide us and show us, as examples, that we too can fulfill our own passions and desires. If you believe in something, then see it through. Nothing is really impossible, sometimes just difficult. Terry and Chris followed their dream. Maybe for most of us it wasn't possible, but for them it was just difficult at times."
—*Tom Schepers, Vietnam veteran, awarded a Purple Heart and a Bronze Star, and walked across the United States to honor veterans of World War II.*

"Sometimes the human body can provide that extra something that a person may need in order to accomplish his or her goals in life. Terry had that extra something. He and his son, Chris, had a dream and whether impossible or not, Terry was going to make his dream come true. We all need to believe in our dreams and know that dreams do come true. We just have to believe."
—*Dr. Tim Rajtora, M.D., an internal medicine specialist and Terry's personal physician.*

"You can grow up to be a person of integrity, knowing right from wrong and acting on it, telling the truth, accepting responsibility for your mistakes, learning from those mistakes, and treating others the way you would want to be treated. Good people trying to do the right thing is what makes our country great. Our everyday heroes are the ordinary citizens who run their own extraordinary daily marathons like Terry and Chris."
—*Coleen Rowley, a Minneapolis-based FBI agent, named one of Time magazine's three "Persons of the Year" for 2002 for her handling of the investigation of convicted terrorist Zacarias Moussaoui.*

"For our lives to be productive and rich with opportunity, we need to have the passion and determination that Terry has to cultivate our dreams and believe in ourselves. Terry ran the first daily marathon to show us it can be done, now with his example and direction we too can run our own marathons and reach our own dreams."
   —Angela Brown, syndicated columnist, triathlete and 29-time marathoner.

"We admire individuals for a variety of reasons: perhaps for their honesty, for their dedication, for their passion for life and how they themselves can be of help to others, for their sincerity, or perhaps for their heartfelt belief that we are all brothers and sisters and trying, in some small way, to make that a reality. That is who Terry is and that, I believe, is why and how he was able to run his 2,000 miles to Atlanta. Everyone told Terry it was humanly impossible but Terry had a dream and he knew that dreams can and do come true. He fulfilled his dream to run to Atlanta and to tell whoever would listen that they too could run their own marathons ... and be successful."
   —Jesse Overton, president of SkyTech, Inc.

"Terry and Chris Hitchcock - You prove that one does not find – but makes the chemistry of success. What stars! ... Your class act demonstrates that with desire, dedication and determination the stage can be set for a joy-full life that plays out with dramatic benefits!"
   —Dale L. Anderson, dramatologist, board certified surgeon, holistic physician, speaker and author of "Never Act Your Age".

"I believe that the one of the best gifts we can give one another is the gift of compassion. Terry Hitchcock exemplifies that belief. Through his depth of compassion, he has championed young and old alike by his incredible achievements. ... Through his dedication to fight for what he believes in, let us all be inspired to do the same ... especially when it comes to the good of our children."
   —Patty Peterson, Jazz singer extraordinaire

"However we manage our lives, however we place our values, we need to always be mindful of the importance of self-management – know thy self, be in touch with feelings and learn how to best coach yourself so you can better manage others. Terry and his son Chris are incredible examples of first coaching oneself and then handing off to others so that they too can best manage their careers and lives. ... In managing our lives, we can see dreams come true and impact those around us in a positive and meaningful manner."
   —Tom Gegax, co-founder, chairman emeritus and former chief executive officer of Tires Plus.

"The day begins with the possibility to make it everything you want. The same goes with each week, year and lifetime. It is a canvas on which you can create whatever you would like. Terry and Chris have done so much while paying no attention to what other people's ideas are of what could or couldn't be done. Absolutely commendable in today's society of suppression, invalidation and victimization. The only way to live life is to get out there and live. The dream is one thing, but to work while you dream is what is necessary."
—*Jennifer Grimm, singer and actress.*

"Whether in business or in our personal lives, we have an opportunity to touch those around us in a positive way. Terry and Chris showed us the way. Each of us can make a difference in the lives of others. It's just a matter of taking that first step. We all can make a difference."
—*Charles M. Denny, Jr., retired chairman and chief executive officer of ADC Telecommunications and a recipient of the Minnesota Center for Corporate Responsibility Distinguished Corporate Citizenship Award.*

"Terry and Chris made certain, in their 2,000-mile trek to Atlanta, that we don't lose sight of this important part of life. Like Terry and Chris, we can all try to do our part to give back and support our children's future. We can all help, maybe not running for 2,000 miles, but in many ways we can and need to give back.'

'Dreams are vital, and so is action, but right now in my country, Iraq, it is a huge struggle to do either. No matter haw hard it is, we must keep dreaming and keep working for the future, though; so that tomorrow our children can have what we most want them to have: the freedom to make their own dreams and shape their own futures."
—*Abbas Mehdi is a Professor of Sociology at St. Cloud State University and previously was Chairman of the Board, Iraq National Investment Commission, Team Leader and Senior Advisor to the Prime Minister's Office and the Council of Ministers, Baghdad, Iraq.*

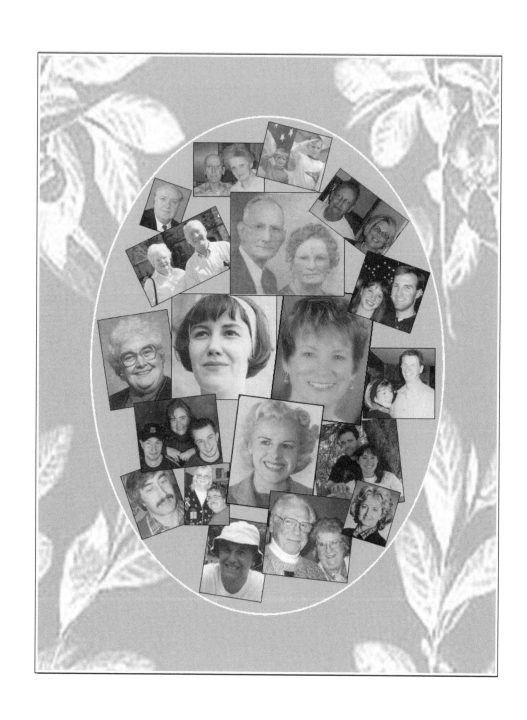

DEDICATION

- **FROM TERRY**

For my children, Teri Sue, Christian, and Jason, and for all children everywhere; Mary Ann and Sue, who provided their love and support and have kept my life light burning; my grandparents, Minnie and Harvey Bolton, who got me through a part of my childhood and especially high school; to my other family members who have continued to believe in me, Mollie and Frank Fecteau; Tom, Stacy, Ryan and Connor Peck; Molly and Ron Mehl; Tim and Lynn Fecteau; Carol and Bill Peck; John and Dorothy Moore; Aleane and Terry White; Estelle and Buddy McWilliams and their sons David, Alexander, Gary and Kevin; to my brother Al and his wife Tina Hitchcock and their children Melanie and Andrew; and to my mother Genevieve "Jean" Campbell.

To Judy Miller, who, with her wisdom, encouraged me to write and to use my gifts; Jerry Vielehr, who taught me to never give up; Sandy Stephens, who knew the real heart of people; Dr. Meghabhuti Roth who showed me how to believe in myself and find inner strength. To the Betsy and Tom Krupp families; to the Woolley, Kronemeyer, Foley, Bramer, Peterson, Marklund, Pope, Fieger, and Turner families, and to the people of North Troy, forever my childhood hometown. And to Peter Jessen, a true and lasting friend.

And to my Heavenly Father who taught me that He would never give me a burden too heavy to carry ... thank you dear Lord.

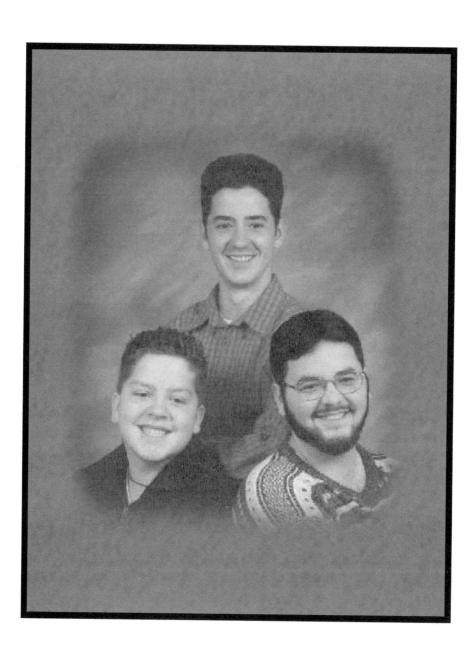

DEDICATION

- FROM PETER

As Terry demonstrates in this book and in his list of people who have positively influenced his life, John Donne was right: "No man is an island"

My dedication, first of all, is to Terry, who has honored me with both his friendship and his invitation to work with him in writing this book. Without the feat of his feet, there would be no book, no film, and no documentary. He and I have worked as consultants together on projects that have taken us across the country to different clients in different settings. I am delighted that he invited me along his run with him, albeit by phone, and in working through the implications and positive consequences as a result of his run in this book.

Second, my dedication is to my college and graduate school professors who enabled me to both grow in knowledge and understanding and taught me to write so that I could express myself clearly. Most importantly, they taught me that to achieve a vision, to attain a goal not obtained before, one has to start with the "is" world, not with the "wish" world that I would like, for you can't get to the "wish" world without starting with the "is" world, with empirical reality. And they taught me the danger of trying to impose on others my "wish" as an "ought" and to be wary of those who would take their wishes and make them other people's "ought." Terry demonstrates this with his run.

Third, my dedication is to my circle of support, my parents, friends and relatives, in church and community, without whom the experience of being a single parent would have been much harder on my three sons.

And so, last but not least, as the last shall be first, my dedication is to my three sons, Eric, Craig and Kyle, now all in their twenties. I raised them within the circle of support above, as a single parent from the time they were ages seven, ten, and twelve. And as a "sandwich-generation caregiver," I simultaneously cared for my parents in their eighties, during the last years of their lives. I experienced the joy of giving, the satisfaction of duty, and the excitement of watching my kids learn to soar, as I too experienced the marathon of the single parent. This is how I understand Terry and why I support his work and efforts. For the joy of my sons I thank God who created our world and gave us abundant life even in single parenting, and for sending these young eagles to share my path, who lightened my load, physically and existentially, emotionally and intellectually.

Life is an adventure to be lived;
not a question to be answered.

—Author unknown

Yesterday is already a dream, and tomorrow is only a vision; but today well-lived makes every yesterday a dream of happiness and every tomorrow a vision of hope.

—Author unknown

Found on a wall in an 1831 farmhouse of
John and Dorothy Moore in
Stanstead, Quebec, Canada

You don't know how much you can really accomplish, until you stand up and try.

—Author unknown

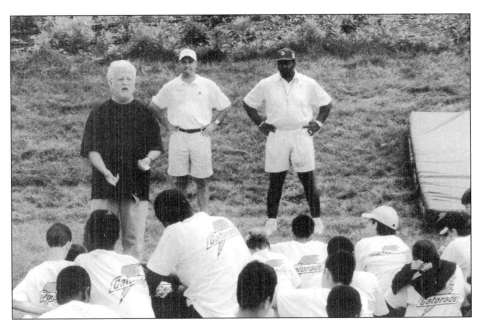

FOREWORD

BY DENNIS GREEN

Former head coach of the Minnesota Vikings and the Arizona Cardinals,
and a youth and community development hero.

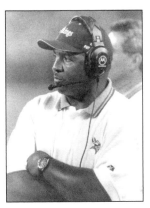

This story is a testament to Terry Hitchcock's personal discipline and dedication, and to his positive perseverance and peaceful patience. Terry is a strong-minded man of courage and stamina who proves that the ordinary guy can do extraordinary things if he has a purpose and the will to make a difference.

For Terry, his dream is to make a difference in the lives of kids everywhere, but in particular in the lives of single parents and their children everywhere. His Olympic-sized effort, which I call the MegaMarathon, focused attention on the struggle that is the everyday marathon of all parents and all children. In our fast-paced world, at a time when children are not a high priority for many, it is an ongoing challenge to build the character of our young people and equip them to build a life they love. Terry believes, and he has persuaded me, that we can provide all kids with a great start in life if we just do some simple things to help the parents we know.

Terry resists attempts to portray him as larger-than-life. He is no media-hungry celebrity athlete – and I've known a few! He is just an ordinary guy achieving extraordinary things because he has a commitment to a purpose larger than himself. Haven't we all needed a helping hand now and then? Aren't we each made a little taller when we bend down to help another? These simple lessons run bone-deep in Terry, and he has my everlasting respect because he had the guts, vision and enthusiasm to put on his shoes and make it happen.

No reader of this book will be able to keep what Terry went through out of his or her memory. Terry is one of those rare people who can enable us to make positive changes in our perceptions, demonstrate to us that hope can be raised and dreams fulfilled, and enable us to see challenges as opportunities to make a difference. In his act of soaring like an eagle, he makes our own spirits soar, raises our sights, and challenges us to make the same commitment to the lives of others.

Terry has been involved in other life marathons as well. He has been an executive in Fortune 500 firms as well as in start-up businesses. He knows the corporate marathon. Terry's background is rich in study and scholarship. He holds a Masters of Business Administration degree, a doctorate in business, and a law degree and honorary degrees. Terry knows the marathon of studying and learning and has taught in graduate business schools, lending academic authority to the authority of experience. Terry established the largest business incubator in the United States adding to his list of over 83 companies that he established or helped establish, creating over 1,513 new jobs. Terry helped establish a technology company that kept kids safe on the Internet. He received the Distinguished Medal of Merit and an American flag from the Republican Presidential Task Force and President Reagan. Terry represented industry and helped establish Grandparents Day, a national holiday, now celebrated in all free countries of the world.

Years ago Terry wrote a book called *American Business: The Last Hurrah?*. For the book he sought insights about what is working and what is not working in our culture from more than one hundred world leaders. He interviewed Gerald Ford, Jimmy Carter, Henry Kissinger, Dean Rusk, Ted Kennedy, Andrew Young, Keijo Saji, foreign heads of state, the leaders of TV networks (NBC, ABC, CBS, CNN), and the heads of international labor unions. He tells me that he learned much about life's marathons from these world leaders – ordinary men and women who also reached deep into themselves to achieve the extraordinary outcomes that make all the difference to other people.

To Terry the marathon is a metaphor for the plain and simple. It represents the preparation, the emotional highs and lows, and the relentless focus and drive needed to accomplish something of merit. This is especially true of those who choose to meet their responsibilities – especially parents.

For Terry and other great sports enthusiasts, a game like football also represents a wonderful metaphor for life. Football players can experience defeat; yet can rise again with heroism to win as in life. Football players need not be perfect, just consistent and committed.

This book offers insights to assist anyone seeking to better understand what motivation is all about. Terry shares with us how to deal with the little-understood phenomenon of depression that comes to many during their lives, especially to athletes after great physical exertion. The story of how Terry successfully completed this run is alternately funny and sad, mundane and profound, and at all times moving and inspiring. Nothing could stop Terry.

One step at a time he brought to life Mahatma Gandhi's observation "What you do may seem insignificant, but it's very important that you do it."

As you travel with Terry on his journey, you will feel a hero awakening within yourself. After reading this book you will not face another day the same way, nor will you doubt your own ability to run your own daily marathons. You will be ready to make whatever Olympic effort is needed for whatever greater purposes you choose.

We need people like Terry Hitchcock and his son Chris. We need them to remind us that we too can achieve great deeds. We can each exceed our reach. We can achieve the grand and great and the simple and beautiful. We need to remember this so we can present the best examples to our kids. Terry reminds us to follow through on our dreams. God will always be there, as He is for Terry, as your coach and co-pilot.

INTRODUCTION

ROBERT GILLIO, M.D.

Founder of InnerLink, LLC, the Lifelong Learning Company.

Terry Hitchcock is a hero to me, but not for reasons you might think. It is true that I am impressed and awed by the fact that he ran seventy-five marathons in seventy-five consecutive days to bring public attention to a cause he believes in. I admire that he rose out of depression after his wife's death, was successful in raising his children and launched a prominent career. As impressive as these feats are, however, it is something else that Terry taught me that elevated him to heroic stature in my eyes. He has given me the gift of realizing that there are heroes all around me. From him I learned to see that it is often the less conspicuous deeds and the small gestures that are truly heroic.

At the hospital where I work, I have noticed that it is not just the near-miraculous surgery that is heroic. The patients are anesthetized during these procedures and care little for the details. The more significant contribution, the one that makes a lasting impression and hastens the healing process, comes from the family member, the volunteer, the nurses' aide or the therapist who holds the patient's hand, cleans up a patient's bed or provides the emotional support so essential yet so misunderstood and undervalued. One can change a recovery prognosis with a simple kindness and a restoration of dignity.

My parents are children of immigrants. As they grew up, they had to deal with issues of poverty, bigotry and war. Their dream was that their children would have a better life than theirs. Everything they did had that singular focus. There were never fancy cars, vacations alone or expensive dinners. Any extra money was put away so that we kids could go to college. They made sure that we went to good schools. Whenever we had trouble during one of our after-school jobs, my father listened patiently. Then, we heard his heroic response: "That's why you are going to study hard and save your money – so you can go to college, so that you don't have to do work like this the rest of your life. If you can dream it, you can achieve it, but you have to work hard to get it."

I also remember my mother's advice. Her simple words have guided me often: "As you make decisions, make sure your family is taken care of first and then do the thing that will make the world a better place." These two heroes of mine supported my decision to become a physician and inventor. Their guiding principles helped me with my patients and subsequently with the patents that developed into three companies whose products and concepts are now distributed worldwide.

More recently, I became frustrated with the plight of a gentleman in our neighborhood. I had known Joe for six years. He was always on the verge of homelessness, yet he still had a positive attitude. He did odd jobs, but he did not believe they were menial, for he always said, "Any job has dignity if it is honest." When this man needed help during a recent Christmas season I talked to a newspaper editor I knew and an article in the paper suddenly had me in the midst of hundreds of heroes. Donations of food and money, as well as offers of employment, poured in. A run-down house that could be fixed up was going to be sold at a silent auction, presenting itself as a wonderful opportunity for this man.

At a family meeting, we sat down and discussed whether our family should consider being one of the bidders on the house. We would have to utilize money that was set-aside for a family vacation and the children's college fund. The kids said, "Go for the house, bid on the house, we don't need a fancy vacation and we'll keep saving for college." As Joe got the keys to his house on Christmas Eve, I realized my kids had experienced the true joy of giving. And I suddenly realized I lived with heroes.

Yes, Terry Hitchcock has done something heroic. He has helped me realize that I encounter heroes every day, in all parts of my life. That is why it is so important to me that his story is read by children, their parents, everyone. I trust his story will open your heart and raise your eyes to new goals beyond the ordinary, beyond which you thought possible. We each can make a difference and we each have a difference to make.

"Big dreams come in little steps. Whenever you get overwhelmed with the big picture, sit down, take a deep breath and plan the next step. At times, it's not a graceful step, sometimes it's not a straight step, but it'll get you foreword and over a tough hurdle one step at a time."

—Polly Letofsky

Walked around the world in her
World Walk for Breast Cancer,
traveling more than
eighteen thousand miles in four years.

CHAPTER 1

PUTTING THE PIECES TOGETHER

This is my story.

I am now sixty-nine years old. At age forty-five a family tragedy changed my life; I became a widower – alone with three children to nurture and a dog to care for.

I didn't know what impact my wife Sue's death would have on me. I was lost in grief and pain. In time, I discovered that Sue's death dramatically changed my outlook on family, work and life. My views on what I should do and could do as a father, provider, executive and human being were pushed onto a new trajectory.

To understand my life and what I have done, you need to understand my motivations. You need to understand how my family life from an early age has shaped who I am and everything I do.

The story begins in Vermont, where I was born. For the most part, I never knew what love or trust was until I was nearly a teenager. My mother had her own burdens to bear, and taking care of a child eventually proved one too many. My absent father was never seen.

My early years were far from stable. I survived my mother's many broken relationships and broken homes. I survived a kidnapping at age 6 by my father. I don't remember much about this incident, but I do know my dad and I traveled by train from Vermont to Boston, where I stayed for many months. Following a knock on the door by Boston police, I was returned to my mother.

The summer before eighth grade my grandparents took me in. I lived in their small home in the farm town of North Troy, Vermont, a community of about four hundred people near the Canadian border. My grandfather Harvey

Bolton worked in a veneer mill. Grandmother Minnie Bolton cooked, baked, and managed a few boarders to help the family make ends meet.

I was on the wrong path in life when I went to live with my grandparents. I was making mistakes and poor choices that could get me in serious trouble. But my grandparents weren't discouraged. They said I could make a difference. They encouraged me. They introduced me to their church. In my short time in North Troy I gained two pillars of strength: my grandparents' home and a church community.

For the first time in my life I learned to appreciate friends and family, and to give and not worry about receiving. I was happy. My grandparents encouraged me to dream, to stand up for what I believe in, and to know God is always with me. It's what I call the Vermont ethic.

Grandpa Harvey died two years before I graduated from high school. I awoke around three in the morning as Grandpa was going downstairs. I heard him say to Grandma Minnie that he wasn't feeling well. I got out of bed and sat on a step halfway down the staircase. I remember him sitting in his favorite chair with a warm glass of milk, and my grandmother was standing beside him. Concerned, and wanting to do something, I walked the rest of the way down the stairs and asked my grandfather how he was feeling. He said fine. He then took a deep breath and died.

Grandpa Harvey made an enormous difference in my life, and in a short period of time. He was my first solid male role model, and now he was gone.

With the loss of my Grandfather's support, Grandma Minnie and I did what we could to keep each other happy and put food on our plates. Grandma Minnie awoke at five every morning to bake cakes, cookies and pies, which she sold to neighbors. I chopped wood, and helped nearby farmers with chores, and I delivered newspapers before going to school. It was hard work. And yet, as poor as we were in material things, we were rich in spiritual things –love and acceptance.

Following high school I joined the Air Force in 1957 where I trained as a medical technician. Eleven months and two days into my service my grandmother became seriously ill and I was given a hardship discharge to care for her. I made Grandma Minnie as comfortable as I could for several months before she died. For a short while I stayed in North Troy, working a number of jobs to pay off her bills.

I didn't realize it at the time, but I had become accustomed to relying heavily on my grandparents for love and guidance. Without them, and the support they had provided, life's complexity overwhelmed me. I briefly tried college at the State University of New York in Fredonia, New York. Instead of studying, I partied and fooled around. I was wasting the tools of life my grandfather had worked so hard to equip me with. I was lost.

I sought refuge in my mother, whom I hadn't seen in five years. We didn't have a solid bond, but in talking with her I began to understand how hard it had been for her as a single parent. I lived with her for a few months in Dunkirk, New York. To support myself I used my Air Force medical technician training to find a job assisting the city's chief pathologist with autopsies, while taking a few evening college courses.

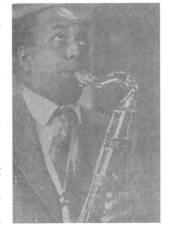

In 1961 I moved to Port Clinton, Ohio, to work as a cost accountant at US Gypsum Company. The new job gave me some spending money and allowed me to buy a convertible – a luxury I prized. I worked hard while also taking night classes at Bowling Green State University. I somehow stumbled into playing saxophone on weekends with my own band as well as with Candy Johnson's band. Candy was a true jazz great who had played with the likes of Count Basie and Bill Doggett. I studied during my lunch breaks and raced to class after work, played saxophone on weekends and, no matter what day of the week, I came home late and exhausted.

FINDING DIRECTION, AND LOVE

I was happy. I had everything a young man could want. Yet, I still felt unsettled. I took a short vacation to travel through Massachusetts, visiting family and friends. I brought my contemplative mood with me, and it changed my life.

While walking on a beach in Massachusetts I met an out-of-place wrinkled old man, who might as well have been a wise Tibetan guru. This stranger saw the searching in my eyes. We talked. He told me to quit my job, sell my car and my possessions, and focus on school, "because no one can ever take your education away from you." At first I thought he was nuts, but as I thought about it I realized he was only telling me what was already in my heart.

I left for home in Ohio with renewed zeal. Whether he was a bum or a prophet, I knew the stranger was right. All the possessions in the world could not take the place of the people I loved. I sold everything and returned to college. I yearned to know more about the way the world works, the way it is, and the ways in which I might apply my gifts to make a difference.

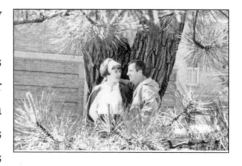

My life changed following this newfound commitment. Shortly after my return to school full time I met a young woman during our training as student advisors. After a few months of playful courtship, Sue and I dated and fell in love. We married in 1967, following my graduation. While Sue finished her Master's in education, I worked and continued going to school at night for a Master's degree in business administration. Our life was full and we were happy. We had great friends. Sue taught students to play piano. I worked hard and found time to play a little racquetball and golf.

We soon had three beautiful children: a lovely daughter and two handsome sons. But, like everyone, we had our worries; both sons incurred life-threatening medical conditions at very young ages. In 1978 Jason gave us a scare when he was ten days old. He needed esophageal surgery to correct an abnormality that forced everything he ate right back up. In 1979 when my older son Chris was three years old, he acquired a life-threatening affliction that produced large brown spots on his chest and stomach. It was an illness I had a hard time pronouncing, much less spelling. I always had to ask Sue to pronounce the name of Chris's disease. Both boys recovered. We felt blessed.

My children's health crises made me reflect on my priorities. I had some success in the business world. I was the typical male in the 1970s, seeking personal fulfillment through experiences in the business world. Although I loved my wife and children very much, I was not always involved in day-to-day activities at home. Instead I spent much of my time at work and writing a book, which required lots of travel as I interviewed the rich and powerful, including Gerald Ford, Ted Kennedy, Henry Kissinger, Margaret Mead, and Andrew Young. I was proud of my accomplishments; my book, *American Business: The Last Hurrah?* had given me some public acclaim.

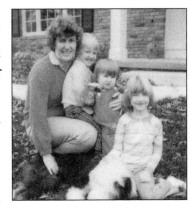

We lived the American Dream. It showed in our marriage, our family, and our lifestyle. We had three children, a sheep dog, a station wagon, and a house in the country. Sue was a teacher and, in addition, found time to teach piano to twenty-four kids every week. She watched over our home and kids while I gave interviews and speeches in front of large audiences around the country.

I left the corporate life for the consulting life. The work was engaging, fun, and fulfilling. Sue and I remained happy, even when faced with a financial crisis caused by a crooked business partner that left me reduced to tears, sitting on a bank floor redeeming our children's savings bonds so we could eat and pay the mortgage.

Through it all, I was surrounded with love and backed by a wife who didn't cast blame, but instead encouraged me and told me it would work out all right. She had enormous faith in God and the peace that faith brings. She helped me attain that grace, too.

I quickly rebounded professionally, taking jobs that often required me to travel. I had few worries and slept well, knowing everything at home was taken care of. I loved the nurturing Sue gave the children and the nurturing she gave to me.

I was learning that everyone needs help in life, whether through encouragement, mentoring, or simply through providing an opportunity. I found this help from my grandparents, business peers, friends and, most of all, from Sue.

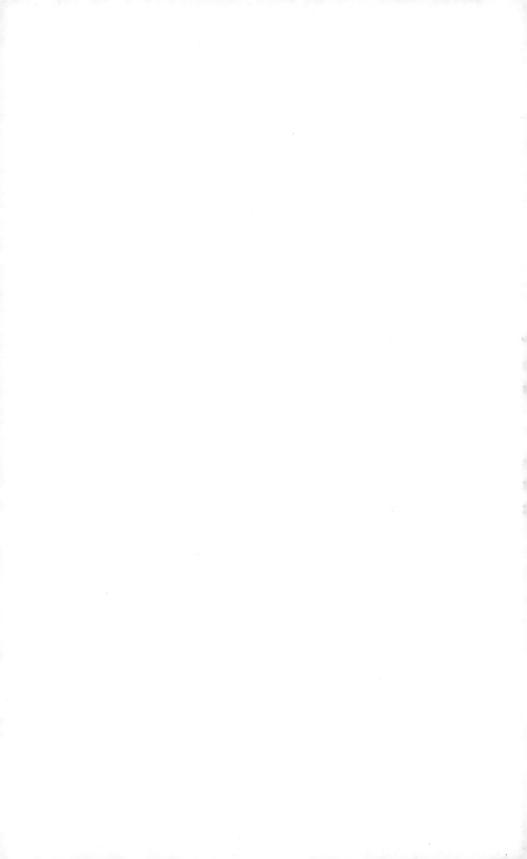

"Life is full of challenges. We need to believe in ourselves and know that we can overcome. Our kids need to believe in themselves and that their dreams can come true. Our kids are our future, our most important investment."

—Tom Petters

Chairman and chief executive officer of
Petters Group Worldwide,
an influential investor in more
than sixty companies, including
Polaroid, Sun Country Airlines and uBid.

CHAPTER 2

NEW PERSPECTIVE

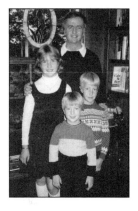

In 1980 I found a great opportunity to spread my wings and gain additional business experience with a fast growing company; we moved to Minneapolis. A few months after we settled into our new home, Sue was diagnosed with breast cancer. Our lives became a hamster wheel of medical tests, chemotherapy treatments, and then cancer remission, before starting over again. Slowly and steadily, the cancer gained strength and ate away at Sue's body.

Through it all, Sue was never concerned for herself. She worried most about the kids and me. She continued to give love and strength to those around her. I felt both blessed and cursed. I felt blessed to have Sue, and cursed that I might lose her.

Sue and I walked down the hospital's halls arm in arm. At times she was connected by intravenous tubes for her chemotherapy treatments. She always greeted her fellow cancer patients with great grace and good humor. I watched Sue, in the midst of her own struggle, encourage them, share smiles with them, and repeatedly tell them they could defeat their own cancers. She had such courage. In my moments of weakness I continued to find strength in her.

Sue was in constant pain as the cancer spread; yet she never complained. By December 1983 her body was so riddled with cancer, she had to walk around home with a bottle of morphine, drinking it like soda pop. I'm not sure if our three kids knew, but I knew; this would be our last Christmas together. Sue and I prayed for strength. We talked and cried together often. During her last months I took a leave of absence from my job and brought in two nurses to care for Sue and the children. Sue insisted on spending her last moments surrounded by those she loved.

A couple of weeks into my leave of absence, I felt I couldn't cope any more. I was physically exhausted. I knelt in prayer and asked God for strength. Kneeling there, as the moon shone through the dining room windows, I felt the Lord providing me with His love. He listened to my tearful cries of pain and I knew then I could again trust Him to carry me.

Through my talks with Sue, and lots of prayer, I came to accept Sue's illness. In the process I became emotionally stronger throughout this time as Sue became physically weaker. We sat on the bed, day and night. Sue and I cuddled and held hands. We felt the meaning of love, unconditionally cared for each other, and took the downs with the ups. Sue remained an inspiration even as she lost weight, withering to around ninety pounds. Even in this weakened state, she still had more mental strength than a football linebacker has physical strength. In God, and in Sue, I found strength.

On her last morning, she asked our youngest son, Jason, to leave for school forty-five minutes early. When we were alone, she squeezed my hand, I kissed her, and she drew her last breath. The marathon of her life ended at age thirty-six.

The following day, where Sue knew I would find it, there was a note addressed to me. Sue's note gave me added courage and strength to move forward with my life and to move forward in caring for our kids. In part it read:

My dearest Terry,

What a time we have had. Who had any idea that when the minister said, for better or for worse, in sickness or in health, it would all happen at once. Thank God it is all over now. I just thought I would let you know that I love you, and admire you. There are not many men who would stick by what we went through. God really blessed me when he gave me you. Tell the children that I will always love them, and I will miss them, but God needed me and I had to go to Him. I wish I had something for the boys, but I can't think of anything. I never did collect baseball cards. We had some wonderful times, honey, and those are the ones to remember, not the last few. I don't think I would have changed a thing in retrospect. Spend time with the gremlins, our wonderful kids. This will be hard for them. The more time you spend together, the easier it may be. I am going to miss you all. This seems so unfair in so many ways, but I know in my heart that God loves us and knows what is best. Be strong, honey, enjoy the gremlins and enjoy life. Get out to meet people, and if you find that right someone, make sure she loves my kids too. Love you forever and two days.

Sue

Sue's letter released me. Without it I would have locked myself in the house and grieved alone. She released me to keep on living and to love again. She gave me a direction outside the events of her death. She wanted me to make certain the kids, ages six, eight, and eleven, were loved, particularly after she had worked so hard to raise them. She wanted to make certain the children remembered to love and care for each other and for others.

The community of support we received after Sue's death helped me and the children get through a very difficult time. Friends and neighbors brought meals or cooked for us in our home. I didn't need to cook for many weeks. In fact, I realized I didn't even know how to cook. I had no experience being a parent at home. Sue had done all of the housework.

COPING ALONE

A few days after Sue's funeral I returned to work to find my office had become the company's new boardroom. My job was gone. The company's board of directors had given me a leave of absence so I would be able to stay home with Sue and the kids during her illness. Instead of being rewarded for years of taking my briefcase home on weekends and working long hours to please whoever was above me on the corporate ladder, I was unceremoniously shown the door.

I had thought I would be welcomed back. I was looking forward to familiar ground, to stepping back into a world where I was confident of my abilities and successful in getting things accomplished even under great adversity. I should have known better. It's called corporate politics and the good old boys got me.

I wanted to scream. I wanted to find a corner and hide. I wanted to hit someone. I wanted to...I wanted to die. Where was God? Where was His all-enveloping, comforting hug? What was I supposed to learn from this?

That night I woke up in a cold sweat, not knowing how to handle the trade-off between my kids and my career. I had to rekindle my career, but now I had more responsibilities at home. Some friends urged me to find family members to raise the kids, which they argued was "women's work." They told me I needed to concentrate on my career so I could provide for my kids "like a man should." But the many hours I spent at home during Sue's illness showed me this was just not right. I could no longer accept that attitude. The thought of it made me angry. I was not going to give up my kids or have them live with someone else when I knew I was capable of taking care of them myself – I just had to figure out *how* to do it.

No matter what else happened in life, I had found meaning in my family. How could I give up my own children? I had helped raise them. I had promised Sue I would take good care of them. Granted, I didn't have many skills with raising children, and, yes, I was scared. I didn't know how to cook and I had no clue about the kids' clothing sizes. What if the kids get sick? Who do I call? What about the kids' piano lessons? How will I manage to earn a living and still be there for them?

Losing my kids would rip out my heart. These were my kids – our kids. They were all I had left after losing Sue. We were still a family. I had grown up in broken homes and terrible situations; I was not going to have my kids experience the same traumas.

I never had a father; my kids were not going to be without a father, too. I wanted them to have as stable a life as possible. I also wanted to *learn* to be a parent, to cook, to tuck them into bed, to read to them, to buy their clothes and know what sizes they wore. All the things that a parent does, I knew I could do. I decided not to move out of town to other job opportunities that were coming my way. I wanted to give my kids stability and love. I knew I could be a great parent.

I wasn't the only one struggling. Sue's death was tough on the kids, too. Teri Sue had to overcome her sadness and anger and her belief that now she had to take care of me. At times Teri Sue's anger led her to scream, and she collapsed on the bed crying. The boys showed their sadness in an increased need for hugs and for someone to wipe away their tears. My oldest son Chris told me two months after Sue's funeral that he felt his mom's presence. Chris said his mom walked down the hall from his bedroom doorway into the master bedroom, surrounded by a brightness of white light. He still feels her presence and guidance and uses this to help him through his personal sadness and tough days.

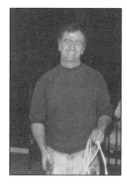

I left behind my corporate identity, with its trappings of a good salary and a plush office. My male friends could not believe I was now cooking supper, buying my children clothes and actually keeping track of their preferences in styles and colors. As I learned how to keep our home clean and prepare meals on time, an orderly transition took place. The kids responded well, getting vanity plates for my car that read DR. MOM. It really fit.

Through it all I struggled. I attended coping and grieving classes. My pastor, Kent Grosser, gave me keys to our church, and I went many times, sometimes at two or three in the morning, just to pray. I occasionally played racquetball, crying as I played. I went to see a psychiatrist to assure myself that I had my head on straight.

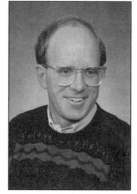

As the kids and I settled into our new lives without Sue, we found there were others we had lost as well. Neighbors who normally visited with us when Sue was alive became distant. Invitations to parties, especially during the holidays, were missing. I feared I soon would have no friends left. A similar thing happened to my children. Their friends were uncomfortable around them. Either no one knew what to say or no one had anything to say. It seemed cold. I was lonely. I found that when Sue died, normal social interaction was more difficult, so perhaps some people just found it easier to ignore me.

Thankfully, some friends stayed, and some did their best to help me through the bad nights and lonely times. My friend Jeff Mangas called me every day at exactly 9 p.m. and we talked about everything, or nothing, until I was ready to say goodnight. Sometimes my good friend Dr. Meghabhuti Roth completed his rounds at North Memorial Hospital, drove twenty miles to my home, and sat all night on my living room floor, talking with me. He taught me self-hypnosis and meditation. He always said I taught him about life and its importance. In truth, he taught me how to live again.

A few months after Sue's death, the kids and I went to a resort in Wisconsin called Northern Pines. The experience stripped away old parts of my life and added new building blocks. For the first time in ages, the kids had big smiles on their faces. They entered a pie-eating contest and became tug-of-war champions, covered with mud from head to toe and ready to go again. We came together as a family. My life, slowly but surely and then completely, became centered on my kids.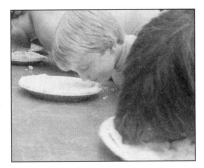

THE FINANCIAL MARATHON

While I was learning to raise three kids, I was also learning to venture out into the business world on my own. I started doing consulting work, and I launched a business incubator with two partners. I wrote more than one hundred business plans for clients and identified various seed money contacts for them. Our incubator soon had more than seventy companies under our wing. We were identified by the Small Business Administration as the largest new-business incubator in the United States. Our dream was to help small businesses in a world where venture capitalists only recognized deals in the millions.

But the financial markets abandoned the mom-and-pop operations and backyard inventors in 1987. We had financed the businesses with our homes and so, when we lost the companies, we lost our homes as well. It was not easy. But we were not looking for security; we were looking for an opportunity to give back to others the many blessings we felt we had enjoyed. We dreamed. We took risks. We lost. We would come back again – that we knew.

The kids and I moved from a six-bedroom house to a small apartment. We stayed together. Dr. Mom prescribed survival. I knew we would overcome and prevail. Life went on. I continued to consult to pay the bills.

I was asked to become president of a young medical company. Seven other business executives and I joined the founder. I was back on my feet with a new house and car, and a more orderly life for my kids. The excitement turned to ashes when we learned that the founder had run up piles of unpaid bills and debt. We all filed for personal bankruptcy.

I then formed my own firm to control my own destiny. I had come full circle. I believed in myself. I knew who I was. I had my values.

I looked for other ways to give back. On one consulting trip I went to The Gambia in West Africa. I saw so much poverty in that country that I decided to provide some food and toys for a few villages. In Minneapolis I helped develop a program called "Reflections," suggested by my friend Dr. Roth, which provided a three-day weekend retreat for seriously and terminally ill people.

Since Sue's death my journey has been a real journey on the path of faith. I learned to be a father. I learned to cook and to take care of three young children. I struggled with depression, financial hardship and the loneliness of being a single parent. But through my struggles I grew. Through our struggles my family grew. God was certainly beside us, and showing not just me, but the entire family, His way. He was there for us; His presence assured us we would be all right.

NOW WHAT?

People often ask me where my story truly began. My marathon started on that dismal day in 1984 when my wife died of breast cancer. Sue was the strength of our family. Sue taught all of us how to hug, to say, "I love you", and to communicate—to be a real family. Since her death, we have continued to grow together and we have tried to be true to her dream. Sue wanted us to be an example of a strong and spiritual family, full of God's love, always believing that there is nothing we can't do if we believe in ourselves.

In 1994 I knew my children were now old enough to participate in my dream. Teri Sue was now twenty-one, Chris was eighteen, and Jason was sixteen. I shared with each of them my dream of helping the more than thirty-five million kids and single parents who, like us, were forced to make do with an incomplete family. All three were very enthusiastic. I wasn't sure I would be able to make a difference.

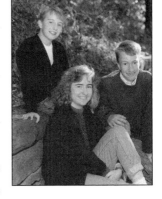

It was my son Chris who came up with the craziest idea: he suggested that the family run to California from Minnesota. I laughed. I was in my mid-fifties and had run only a few ten-kilometer races—where I always came in last. But the more I thought about running long distances the more intrigued I became.

"Life can throw nothing at you that God can't use for your benefit. This is your life. It was carefully drawn up in God's playbook just for you. If you totally trust Him, He won't let your life end one yard short. Terry and Chris trusted in the Lord and were able to cross into the end zone. You can too."

—Les Steckel

Veteran NFL Coach and
President of the Fellowship of Christian Athletes

CHAPTER 3

TURNING ORDINARY INTO EXTRAORDINARY

Chris's suggestion reminded me of one of my heroes, Terry Fox, and his attempt to run across Canada on an artificial leg in 1980. His feat had been etched in my mind as I read the newspaper and followed his progress. See www.terryfoxrun.org.

Terry lost his right leg above the knee because of a bone cancer. At age nineteen he attempted to do the seemingly impossible, to run across Canada from the Pacific Ocean to the Atlantic. His mother used to say he was "average in everything except determination."

Terry did not become despondent or angry over the hand life had dealt him; he grew determined. He retained his sense of optimism and joy of life. The suffering and courage of other cancer patients he came to know while he was in the hospital had moved Terry. He was inspired to run across Canada, roughly five thousand miles, in a "Marathon of Hope" to raise funds for cancer research.

Terry Fox's run lasted about four-and-a-half months before chest pains lead to an examination which showed his cancer had returned – this time to his lungs. He didn't complete his journey, but he inspired millions and raised millions of dollars for cancer research. I was one of those millions of people he inspired.

Like Terry Fox, I wanted to make a difference and pass on a vision of a better world. By now I knew only too well the story of single parents and I wanted to raise the awareness of the plight of single parents and their kids. I knew that just talking about the issue wasn't going to accomplish enough. I knew I needed to share my passion in a tangible way that people could see and feel and follow – just like I had followed Terry Fox so intently all those evenings in 1980.

And so I decided to run from the Twin Cities of Minneapolis and St. Paul, Minnesota, to Atlanta, Georgia, approximately two thousand miles over seventy-five consecutive days. I chose Atlanta because it was where two of my children were born, and as host of the 1996 Summer Olympics, it represented the hopes and dreams of so many young people. In going to Atlanta I would have to run an average of at least twenty-six miles a day – every day – for seventy-five consecutive days.

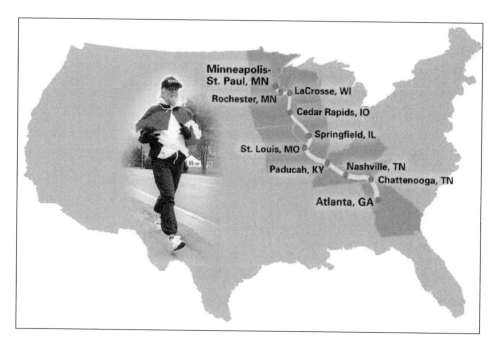

A DREAM IS ONLY CRAZY UNTIL YOU BELIEVE IN IT

The day the idea for the Run was born I began to see all the aspects of my life as a marathon, including the planning and preparation. I had to begin physical training, but I also had to be mentally tough, so I could go the distance.

The first step on the road to my run was to form the *Children Are Forever* foundation to raise funds to help single-parent children and create awareness in the minds of others. I could think of no better way to generate interest than to undertake a Run. The *Children are Forever* foundation's goal, as outlined in its mission statement, was to "support the innocent children of single-parent families" and to "support parents and their children as they deal with the unique frustrations and difficulties of single parenting, including providing such family support as co-op childcare, counseling, and other services/assistance for single parents and their families."

In November 1994, I felt ready; I invited friends to join me for an announcement. Nearly 60 friends came to a neighborhood hotel to hear my announcement of the Run, to learn of my dream, to celebrate this decision with me, and to listen to a description of my plans. I invited them to help me make the dream come true. I then answered their many questions.

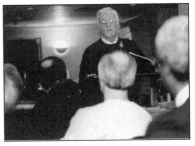

I will always remember that night. No one questioned my sanity – though some would later. I received a lot of support and gained faith that perhaps I had a chance to pull this off. With God and friends at my side, and my focus on the millions of single parents and their kids, I knew I would somehow make it to Atlanta. I planned to take that first official stride to Atlanta on May 2, 1996. Then I would take the next stride, and the next stride, and the next, until my hundreds of strides turned into thousands of strides. My plan was to run through more than one hundred towns and cities along the way, arriving seventy-five days later on July 15, 1996.

My decision to run the MegaMarathon was not based on any prior running experience. Before now I was never a runner. My passion had always been for racquetball – in a good week, I played three or four times. I never ran as a hobby or as part of a workout regimen.

However, in my life it is not failure or even loss that is most painful, but rather regret. I have been presented many opportunities I did not take out of fear, fatigue, or simple confusion. But, in spite of the missed opportunities, suffering and hardship in my life, I have much to be thankful for. I thought of the Run as a way to not only help my own children and all children learn how to best use their gift of life. I wasn't going to let this opportunity, this Run, go by.

As I looked at my strapping sons Jason and Chris, then seventeen and nineteen, and my daughter Teri Sue, then twenty-two, I wanted to leave a legacy of living life fully, placing family first, and not letting anything stand in the way of family. I grew up with the pain of broken homes, shattered dreams, and sadness. Misfortune in the guise of cancer robbed my kids of their mom just as they began growing into their own. My kids grew up in a single-parent home, as more than half of kids do today.

This is why I decided to try to make a difference in the lives of other single-parent families and children everywhere. I wanted to leave a lasting memory for my kids. I wanted to remind them to be thankful for what they have and to know that their mom still lives within them. She is a guardian angel, watching over them, silently standing guard as they go about the marathon of daily living.

Can just one person make a difference? I knew it to be true. Each person who participated as a support team member on this Run made a tremendous individual difference in the lives of many others. We set a goal, committed to our goal, and then acted on that commitment.

PUBLIC AWARENESS MEANS GREATER SUCCESS

As I prepared for seventy-five marathons in seventy-five consecutive days, I prepared not only for the physical marathon, but also learned to articulate the marathon as a metaphor for single parenting. I know from experience that we are all, in the final analysis, ordinary, though we are all capable of doing something extraordinary. The extraordinary person, above all else, brings vision, enthusiasm, and perseverance to their task. In a word, the extraordinary just "do."

But even a great idea with a powerful vision does not guarantee success. Mother Theresa labored in obscurity for forty years before her story was told by a visiting news team. Publicity did not add to the value of her work but it made it accessible to others, and they became inspired to do likewise. In this way, the media can be an important tool. I also hoped to inspire action to help single-parent families — and I wanted to use the Run and the media to do this.

In my mind, the path to helping single parents and their children was quite simple: Define the problem, put a face with it so that people can relate, then generate a discussion about it that will lead to a consensus approach to solving the problem. It was easy to say, much harder to do.

IN THE ARENA

I have had setbacks and misfortunes in my life, successes and failures, and gains and losses. That is part and parcel of ordinary life. But now, I dared to enter another arena. I hoped an extraordinary feat, my Run, would raise awareness of the plight of single-parent families everywhere.

One man whom I admire did just that. This asthmatic young man struggled to overcome being a weakling. As a myopic, bespectacled young man he dug deep within himself and found strength to overcome physical infirmities. He stood tall in terms of exercising his enthusiasm and perseverance in order to make a difference. This young man was Theodore Roosevelt. Roosevelt became President of the United States in 1912. He was the "trust buster" who challenged the era's rapacious monopolies and enabled new people to get into the capitalist game. His bespectacled visage is one of the four honored on the face of Mount Rushmore, and the only one from the twentieth century.

In the following speech in Chicago in 1899, Teddy urged us to "dare mighty things," and to get "in the arena."

> *"Far better it is to dare mighty things, to win glorious triumphs, even though checkered by failure, than to take rank with those poor spirits who neither enjoy much nor suffer much, because they live in the gray twilight that knows not victory nor defeat.*
>
> *"It is not the critic who counts, not the man who points out where the strong stumbled, or how the doer could have done better. The credit belongs to the man who is in the arena, his face marred by dust and sweat and blood, who strives valiantly, who errs and falls short again and again: there is no effort without error.*
>
> *"But he who tries, who knows the great enthusiasms, the great devotions, who spends himself in a worthy cause, at best knows the triumph of achievement, and at the worst, fails while daring. His place shall never be with those cold and timid souls who know neither victory nor defeat."*

Not only words to live by – words to live extraordinarily by.

"We know that if we can instill in children the dreams of extending themselves to achieve in life, teaching them will be easier than when they don't have dreams. Terry's story should be read to every school child in America, and throughout the world, to help them understand the power of holding onto and following their dreams."

—Richard Barbacane

Educator and Former President of the National Association of Elementary School Principals

CHAPTER 4

AND SO IT BEGINS
WITH TRAINING

For the single parent every day is a marathon and there is rarely a training course. It's nearly impossible to know how difficult solo parenting is until it's a reality. With the Run, I was the Single Parent as Marathon Runner: I exercised the arts of parenting and perseverance.

The target start date for the Run was May 2, 1996. Seventeen months before that date, I began the long journey to put my body in shape to accomplish what many people (or more precisely, everyone) said was physically impossible. Doctors, runners, and friends told me it was not humanly possible to run a marathon, 26.2 miles, for seventy-five consecutive days. To prepare myself for the ordeal I combined the outward journey to prepare my body with an inward journey to prepare my mind.

I chose Scott Meier as my trainer. He was the best, and he had to be. I wasn't eighteen years old. For that matter, I wasn't twenty-, thirty-, or even forty-something. I was fifty-six years old when training commenced, and I would be fifty-seven when I left for Atlanta in May. Scott is a wonderful and gifted trainer. He is quiet, yet intense. He has all the qualifications of a professional trainer – the academic degrees, the life experiences – and is a runner 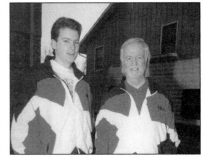 himself. Scott pushed me to and beyond my limits without my even knowing it. If I fell down I got up because Scott was there and I didn't want to disappoint him. He gave me plenty of room to make mistakes, and I was driven by some inexplicable desire to please him, to prove to him that I could take that next step. His judgment was uncanny. Scott possesses an innate gauge for progress; he knew exactly how hard to push, never forcing me to the point of quitting, but never letting me take it easy.

Scott and I met almost every day for seventeen months. We plotted our course, planned my workout schedule, and attacked "The Mountain." We called it The Mountain because my training encompassed much more than just running. I needed to be strong on all fronts to survive all elements. I planned to run more than twenty-six miles each day for seventy-five consecutive days, and I needed the ability to overcome any obstacle or problem for that stretch of time. Scott taught me Robert A. Schuler's image of running: running is like climbing a series of mountains. If you can't run over them you run around them or tunnel through. Every problem is its own mountain. When you encounter one you visualize yourself climbing, circling, or tunneling. Then, you execute. Each mountain becomes a positive experience, a gold mine yielding great riches. Long tasks are accomplished by turning the pain of effort into the gold of satisfaction that comes with an accomplishment – that gold is the currency of successful runs.

I would find out on my Run just how true that is. The long Run became a series of smaller Runs to achieve, and smaller Runs were feats I could cope with. In order to finish the complete Run I could not allow myself to focus on the long-term goal itself – I had to defeat each smaller segment, knowing through my planning that the succession of accomplishments led to the larger prize.

I lifted weights, stretching until every bone and muscle in my body felt out of place. Then I did it again. I did short runs of five or six miles at a time. During my training, my cholesterol dropped from 255 to 155, and my resting pulse fell from 69 to 51. My major physical problem during the entire training period was my right Achilles tendon. It felt like a sharp knife was sticking me in the ankle day and night. I climbed the Achilles Mountain every day and questioned my desire to continue training with nearly every step.

Besides the sore Achilles tendon, I had trouble with my feet. At times running any significant distance seemed as impossible as people had warned me the Run would be. Nevertheless, Scott and I ran and trained for almost a year and a half in all kinds of weather. We ran in rain and snow, hot weather and cold, it didn't matter. Sometimes the temperature was twenty degrees below zero, with a wind chill added to the bitterness. I often returned from a run with ice hanging from my eyebrows and my beard. But we rarely decided it was "too cold" for practice. Weather in Minnesota can change in a heartbeat and I knew I would encounter all kinds of weather over the two and a half months of the Run. Likewise, with two thousand miles to travel I had to anticipate all kinds of terrain. Thus, we ran various back roads and highways. We ran more hills than I wish to ever climb again.

Scott also sprinkled throughout my running schedule various weight and strength training routines, as well as water exercises. At various times one knee or the other would be so pained I had to stop. Running in deep water relieved the pressure on my knees and rehabilitated them quickly so I could resume running. I knew I couldn't miss a single day – and I trained every day of the week – if I wanted to continue building stamina, endurance, and strength.

Interestingly enough, the Achilles problem that had persisted for more than a year of training vanished three weeks into the Run and never returned. Throughout the entire 2,000 miles I felt my body heal itself. During training and through the first ten days of the Run, I experienced sharp pains in my left hip and both knees and ankles. However, after that first ten days, these seemingly chronic conditions slowly vanished. The remaining eight and one-half weeks held only dull pain and low-grade discomfort at least most times.

I questioned the sanity of the Run at times. Throughout the training period it seemed like I had been running and training for a much longer time. Then I considered all the kids and parents struggling with their daily marathons and I knew I would get through somehow. Just the image of crossing the finish line in Atlanta filled me with a rush of exhilaration that can only be understood by those who act on the urge to accomplish a great task.

I had a strong faith in myself, a strong faith in God, and a strong faith in all the people who came forward to put together the pieces of this puzzle. The faith I had in my community of supporters felt like the faith I imagine people had for each other during old-fashioned barn raisings, when the entire community came together for the benefit of a single family. Their faith was well placed and so was mine. Each member of the Run community gave help knowing his or her turn to receive help would follow. There were moments when I might not have made it if not for the friends and supporters taking turns to raise me up. At different stages of the Run, they literally showed up to give me a hug, to lift my spirits, and to deliver an infusion of care and belief. For example, an expert from Stillwater, Minnesota, introduced me to a specialized massage technique, rolphing, which helped me through some very painful times. Rolphing was a very, very deep massage, all the way to the bone, and it was painful; yet it did the trick. Her compassion, generosity, and support enabled me to commence the Run.

And certainly, God was the ultimate team member. He carried me often along the road to Atlanta. Two thousand miles is a long way for any man or woman, but nothing to God. I was comforted when I envisioned a single pair of footprints in the sand – God's footprints, with me in His arms.

The training itself became a metaphor for the Run, for preparation and conditioning and overcoming the summit of self. Once my spirit was truly willing, my flesh would have to be equally capable. As Scott often phrased it, the preparation became the highest mountain. If I could climb this one I could climb any I would encounter along the way. By the end of training my body would be ready to perform the feats my mind demanded of it.

Before I started the actual Run in May of 1996 I could never run more than six miles at any one time. But with Scott's help and the support of many others, I had learned to climb the small hills and knew I could face the numerous personal mountains along the way. I knew there would be many to come, both physical and otherwise. I had to raise funds, coordinate the people handling the various preparations, and make public appearances. Throughout it all, of course, I had to run.

I was nearly halfway through the training and my body had never been so well tuned. I was already taking better shape than I had been in for years. I knew I would never have the chiseled physique of a young athlete, but I needed to reduce my cholesterol, gain muscle, lose fat, and build endurance – especially in my legs. I anticipated it would take more than five million strides to get to Atlanta within the seventy-five days and I wanted to make every one of them. So I pushed myself through every ache and pain imaginable. I coughed up blood. I cried myself to sleep with muscle cramps that refused to go away. I dealt with the excruciating pain as best I could, and when I needed them, my friends and supporters were there to help. I slowly lost fat, gained endurance, and built strength. I might never be a young athlete, but I was well on my way to becoming an athlete who could do what everyone said was impossible.

Then I had a heart attack.

"The daily marathons we run each day are filled with excitement and challenge. One such challenge is the plight of our kids and their families. Like Terry and his son Chris, we all need to learn from our daily marathons and to believe in our dreams."

—John A. Kelley

Twice won the Boston Marathon ('35, '45)
and is a two-time Olympian ('36, '48).

He also has run in a record sixty-one Boston Marathons

CHAPTER 5

HEART ATTACK MOUNTAIN

Scott told me the chest pains and squeezing sensation were signs of a heart attack. I didn't believe him. I thought they were just symptoms of strain. I was wrong. I went from training to intensive care, where I stayed for ten days. The doctors confirmed I had a heart attack. I couldn't believe this would happen while my body was becoming better and better conditioned. It seemed unfair, to say the least. I had spent more than six months conditioning, following a regimen of self-improvement that my body should have appreciated. Instead, my body betrayed me.

And yet, this was just one more mountain to climb. It turned out to be the most incredible part of my training, not because it was life threatening, but because it was life focusing, life transforming, and life affirming.

I had heard that many people view a heart attack as a wake-up call, reminding them of the precious gift of life and serving as an eye-to-eye encounter with their inner core. They come to an understanding of how they really want to invest their time and life and how they want to be remembered if the heart attack actually proves fatal. My heart attack similarly impacted me. It renewed my resolve and made me want to double my efforts. I stopped complaining. I refused to be deterred from my dream. The heart attack became another positive turning point. It further spurred my commitment to help kids and strengthened my resolve to help single-parent families. I was determined to turn this mountain into an opportunity to redouble my efforts. Perhaps.

My family rallied around me and around each other. I temporarily was no longer the center of strength for the family. Jason had shied away from hospitals since his mom died, but he visited me and was very considerate. I knew he was uncomfortable as we talked in my hospital room, but he was concerned and wanted to share his love with me, showing me his artwork and talking about his music. Chris, on the other hand, was past the point of being uncomfortable in a hospital and wanted to be with me as my friend. He told me he loved me. Any parent can understand the significance and healing power of hearing that phrase from a son or daughter. Teri Sue gave me special cards and said all the right words, too. My kids had learned well.

My cardiologist, Dr. Lyle Swenson, said there was no question that my heart attack was serious, but not as serious as it could have been. He told

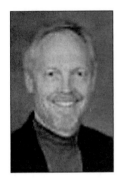

me that a heart attack centered in the bottom portion of the heart is the least life threatening. That was where my heart attack occurred. To prevent another, I was given an angioplasty to open a closed artery. Tests taken afterward showed that my attack was the kind for which exercise promoted healing. Thus, my dream was positive not only in terms of its vision, but also in terms of my own physical healing. *Whether* I would run was not a question; the only question was how close I could come to my desired May start date. It was still seven or eight months away. I was now just half way through my training and determined to let nothing stand in my way.

As I lay in my hospital bed in the intensive care unit I told Dr. Swenson that I still wanted to fulfill my dream of running to Atlanta. He was shocked. He could see I was dedicated and just a little bit stubborn. Rather than resurrecting the old chorus of "It's impossible," he decided to do all he could to help. He gave me the advice I needed to return to my training. I promised all the doctors on the team that I would keep in contact with them so they could monitor my progress and address any physical problems that might arise.

My good friend Dr. Meghabhuti Roth pointed out that there was little margin for error as I pushed my body to its limit every day. It was imperative to drink every twenty minutes without fail. If I became thirsty, it was too late. Thirst meant I had already gone too far and needed to find an emergency room immediately. It also meant I had gone over the edge physically and needed intensive care. I never forgot that advice. A day never started during the run without lining up the water bottles. Dr. Roth had already seen me through some of the darkest nights of my life when Sue died, now, once again, his advice would keep me alive.

"Terry possesses extraordinary vision and demonstrates extraordinary commitment for the causes he champions. Within these, children are paramount and he continues to perform at a marathon pace in everything he does, every single day. I am amazed at the perseverance that I see in Terry. Years ago, I did a painting that shows an eagle flying high above the clouds, bathed by the sun. I called it Rise Above The Story. Terry is the personification of that eagle. Sure, there are storms but he rises above them and finds the sunshine!"

—Mario Fernandez

A world-renowned painter and sculptor born in Havana, Cuba, imprisoned for political dissent at age sixteen.

In 1965 Mario found freedom in the United States.

CHAPTER 6

FROM MOUNTAINS TO WALLS

My friend Dr. Meghabhuti Roth is a marathon runner himself. He explained to me that long distance runners face two walls. The first is known and easier to prepare for. The second occurs when you push yourself beyond human limits.

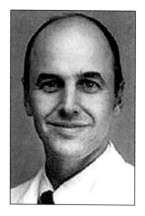

Most marathon runners talk about and have experienced the first wall, which they hit somewhere around the twenty-mile mark. However, as my doctors pointed out, this experience is not universal and can be avoided with the right preparation. It's a physical thing; the body runs low on glycogen, making you feel certain you cannot go on. If you don't prepare properly you experience it; if you prepare properly, you probably won't. The key to getting through this wall is consuming plenty of carbohydrates, including liquid carbohydrates and sports drinks. However, because my physical ordeal would extend for seventy-five consecutive days, I had to be especially well prepared. I would not be taking the usual rest periods after each segment. After each marathon, I would run another the next day, and the next, and the next. Would I hit this wall each day?

Runners seldom, if ever, experience the second wall. It's not necessarily an obstacle that those who run a very long distance must get through to be successful. It may come during the run, or it may occur after completion. Contributing to the second wall is something all marathoners suffer to some degree after a run: delayed onset muscle soreness, or DOMS. Tests show it is best not to run for a week after a marathon—a fact that worried all of my doctors. I would not be resting, so even if I were prepared for the first wall, I would somehow have to push past the compounded soreness layered each day on my muscles. With the weight of many layers of DOMS upon me, what mental walls awaited me?

The second wall is sometimes experienced as the let down at the end of a run. It is part of the unique emptiness long-distance runners experience. Those who have gone through it believe it is something only another long distance runner can understand. I came to see it as a metaphor for achievement, for refusing to settle for a seat on the sidelines. I saw it as seizing an opportunity to play in the arena. These, among many other thoughts, helped keep me going during the preparation and later during the Run.

The let down sometimes manifests as outright depression. I was warned that it is impossible not to experience at least some everyday depression and possibly a great deal of it, given the incredible nature of an effort like this. Post-marathon depression is not unlike the postpartum depression some women feel after childbirth. For both the runner and the expectant mother, life revolves around the planned event. When it is over, the concentration and resolve are no longer needed and emptiness remains. The fulfillment of having achieved a long-sought goal can quickly be replaced by a loss of significance, a hollow sense of, "What now?"

And this is after just *one* marathon. I planned to run seventy-five consecutive marathons. It can take several weeks to recover from a single instance of second wall depression – I wondered how many weeks or months I would need to recover after potentially experiencing it seventy-five times.

According to my doctors, it is natural to experience "everyday depression." There is a significant difference between depression of this type, which affects twenty-five to thirty percent of the population, and clinical depression, which afflicts only seven percent of the population at any given time. Although studies show that one-third of our population will suffer clinical depression at some point in their lives, the good news is that most episodes last only three to six months and nearly half of the afflicted recover with no recurrence.

So, as I was to end the Run in July, the worst-case scenario would have me recovering fully by no later than the end of the year.

Depression is best dealt with by taking time off to relax and recharge the physical and mental batteries. Various doctors suggested to me that depression need not necessarily be treated with anti-depressants. Setting and acting on new goals are effective healing measures to combat depression, as well as engaging in "self-talk" – cognitive restructuring. Self-talk is the conscious creation of positive statements of self-affirmation to counter any negatives entering the mind. It's a neatly mathematical philosophy: offsetting the negative with the positive brings one back to equilibrium.

"As Terry's doctor, I could only stand back and be amazed. Training. Heart attack. More training. The Run. Bone fractures. He completed his impossible run. Seventy-five marathons in seventy-five consecutive days. A great story. A great inspiration to all."

—David Thorson, M.D.

Sports Medicine Specialist

CHAPTER 7

VISION

I was convinced that I could run to Atlanta even though I had a serious heart attack. I felt it could be done; I was going to give it my best effort. Children and single parents were too important not to somehow share their plight.

During the 1996 Olympic Games my heart was captured by Kari Strug when she executed her vault with an injured leg, capturing the gold medal for the U.S. women's gymnastics team. This amazing moment in Olympic history occurred only weeks after my Run. As I sat and watched young Kari on television, I thought I knew what she had been through. She had jumped for her team. She had jumped for her country. She had a purpose. Regardless of what went through her mind as she started that painful journey to the vault, millions of people witnessed her driving through the pain to achieve what many may have thought impossible.

I, too, had a purpose. I intended to run for my team: single parents and their children. To be sure, my story and Strug's were marked by contrast. The achievement of Strug's youth and talent took place on the grandest of stages, under the gaze of hundreds of millions of eyes. Mine took place in more humble settings across our nation's heartland, during a more mature period of my life. It just goes to show that life-altering achievements can occur at any age, in any place.

This is where vision comes in. Some people say they just aren't into "the vision thing." And yet, who but those with vision can withstand the pain of struggle? Who but those with vision will persevere? From the vision comes the desire to fulfill the vision. My vision motivated me to determine specific goals for myself, then inspired the planning and execution to meet those goals. I couldn't have done it without a passionate vision. Excitement and motivation are created by vision – the ability to see the possibilities of the future.

The mind controls the body. The key to a body's performance is the mind believing in the success of the outcome. The fact that no one has accomplished a task before hardly makes it impossible – just look at Sir Edmund Hillary. When he first suggested climbing Mt. Everest, people laughed. It was impossible. Why? Simply because that feat had yet to be achieved. Many had tried; all had failed. Pessimism led to ridicule when Hillary's first few attempts failed. But he kept trying. When he finally succeeded in 1953 he was the man of the hour. He appeared on magazine covers and was invited to many speaking engagements. And since his groundbreaking achievement, the impossible has been accomplished more than 400 times.

Sir Roger Bannister was the first runner to break the four-minute mile in 1954. Again, the feat was considered impossible. It was the threshold across which the human body simply could not pass – until Bannister passed it. Since then, the impossible has been achieved regularly in every major world meet, on many college track teams, and on a few high school teams as well.

In both of these cases the impossible was a mental state, a manifestation of groupthink. Hillary and Bannister stood out because they didn't dwell on their shortcomings. Rather, they showed the world they could achieve with what they had. They showed that impossible and possible are only concepts, reality lies in the attempt and the achievement. They didn't dwell on impossible, and neither did I. I clung tenaciously to the idea of the possible. I found that as I did so the circle of what was possible expanded to include success.

You must have strong faith to stand up to critics and their conventional wisdom.

I was also intrigued by the idea that support from others greatly influences health and healing and often enhances the development of mental toughness. More and more the research indicates this is so. Nick Hall has dubbed it, "Vitamin S" or what I call social support—or just plain hugs.

Nick is a psychoneuroimmunologist. He has done pioneering research in the interrelationships between emotions and health. His book *Mind Body Interactions and Disease* deals with healing and the mind. I needed all the Vitamin S I could get, and thankfully, I was given plenty. First and foremost among the people providing Vitamin S were my family: Teri Sue, Chris, and Jason, and of course, my dog Charlie, a white boxer who was my training buddy. In addition to the expert guidance from Scott, I had excellent ongoing advice from my doctors and inspiring support from many volunteers and well wishers.

Among the many friends and volunteers who provided support, one stands apart from the rest: J. Marie Fieger of Neimer Fieger & Associates, one of the top public relation's professionals in the Twin Cities and the Midwest. She gave us thousands of public relations hours to make certain we were successful in drawing attention to our endeavors. She and the army of volunteers and supporters she coordinated were exactly what I needed during the pain and setbacks of training. Their support would carry over in my mind 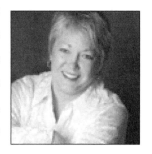 during the Run. J. Marie was the backbone of this MegaMarathon in so many ways. Her tenacity to make certain everything was done and done on time was always present. She was totally dedicated to my dream as was her firm. She was our angel. She was magic to so many of the volunteers who perhaps even questioned, now and then, how I was even going to get a few days or a few weeks out from the Twin Cities before this trek would end abruptly. She was our point person. J. Marie was our heartbeat back in the Twin Cities. Until the heart attack I gave little conscious thought to my health. I assumed I would be healthy because I always felt good. Besides, through my training I was rapidly progressing from good to better. I never thought I would find myself flat on my back with severe pain that refused to stop, or that I would be connected by tubes to machines that kept blinking vital signs at me. It was frightening, but I couldn't let fear stop me. With the support from my team and my community, both medical and personal, I reaffirmed my commitment to my vision, overcame my fear, and moved forward.

Training the body is much easier than training the mind. Although the mind and body are one, united, they are also separate. Despite conditions such as the second wall, the mind, as far as we know, influences the body more than the reverse. As I prepared for the Run I found that my mind, not my body, had the upper hand and was in control. I had to keep negative thoughts out and positive thoughts in. Martin Luther once said he couldn't keep the birds from flying over his head but he could keep them from making nests in his hair. So too, it was with me. I could not keep negative thoughts from entering my mind, especially when they were uttered aloud before me by skeptics, but I could refuse to let those thoughts stay. Through my training I came to understand the difference between looking at people as minds with bodies, rather than bodies with minds.

Skeptics come in all different shapes and sizes. I met many people who smiled with me and then laughed as I passed. I can't really blame them. Who would believe my body, with its silver hair, would take me as far as it did? Running in the league of seasoned runners who had three percent body fat was a joke. Sometimes I was lucky to make the next hill without having my less-than-svelte body cry out in pain. I'm sure I was seen as a joke at times, or at least I felt like I was. What was I trying to prove? My close friends knew of my determination and stubbornness. But the rest? They said, "Why bother?" "Who cares?" "Why would anyone keep doing that to his body?" or "You will never make any real difference, nothing will change." The hindrance of skeptics can be very damaging, so I made it a point to not let those birds nest in my hair.

Through all of this preparation I was still a father and a single parent for my three children. I needed and wanted to meet their needs. Having to parent them helped distract me from focusing on the discomforts and pains of training. The Run would soon commence and then be over, but their lives would go on. By remembering my long-term role as father, and focusing on the short-term goals of raising children, I was able to let my mind join forces with my body to keep me focused and on-task.

Another struggle for my mind was to find inward peace when there was outward turmoil. This was not a sponsored Run. Big bucks did not stand behind it, although friends familiar with my Run lined up nutritional and running equipment, as well as clothing donations from manufacturers. The Run was mainly financed by money I borrowed and through fundraisers held prior to and during the Run itself. Often the funds were driven to us so we could make needed purchases en route. In this metaphor for life, this mirrored the daily economic marathon of many single parents living paycheck-to-paycheck or even day-to-day. In a society with so many dual-income families, a single-income family has a hard time both socially and economically. When a spouse dies or a couple divorces, the parent with the children is too often left with less money and certainly less time than before.

During the training period and during the Run itself I was indeed running a dual marathon: the daily run to earn an income and support my family, and the training for and execution of the MegaMarathon. I was still a management consultant and still needed to spend time with my family. Clients had to be served. My business partner, Zak Manuszak, was great at keeping everything together. He made sure that Hitchcock Company remained a viable consulting firm and that our clients were not only served but served well.

As my training continued I felt my body, my emotional state, and my spiritual outlook grow stronger and more positive. This progress was sustained by several people who helped me participate in activities I loved as well as activities I needed. Racquetball is my favorite sport; I could play it for hours when I was in shape. Before training, I played racquetball a couple times each week but, like many people, I was a couch potato the rest of the time. I had a variety of excuses for my sedentary life, but the fact remains that I wasn't pushing myself physically. With the Run ahead, I had to stay off the couch and offer no excuses. My physical survival was at stake and the success of the Run hinged upon my personal ability. For the first time in years, probably since American Legion ball and in college, I came alive with new energy and a new outlook. And as my body became conditioned, so did my mind.

No matter what the doctors, major league runners, or some friends said, I was going to run (or crawl if I had to) an average of more than twenty-six miles each day for seventy-five consecutive days. My personal mantra became, "Watch out Atlanta, here I come." I had to follow the same advice I gave clients: maintain a positive attitude, accentuate the positive and minimize the negative. I found if I read inspirational materials each day and then meditated on the messages as I trained I could take on anything. I was determined to run a good race. I was determined to make it all the way.

In *Man's Search for Meaning*, Victor Frankl described his discovery of the final freedom while confronted with the reality and horror of living in Nazi concentration camps in World War II. He was stripped of everything, including human dignity. As his captors forced him to stand naked in the cold, he attained this insight: he could only control his attitude and his reactions. Through this undeniable ownership he was able to find the power of forgiveness and the power of positive thinking, no matter how severe and traumatic the situation. This insight meant a lot to me during both my training and my Run.

Through my vision I was convinced the Run could be done.

"This is an unbelievable story of a person who wanted to make an important difference in the lives of children and families everywhere. Terry Hitchcock is a real hero."

—Sandy Stephens

Quarterback for the 1960 University of Minnesota National Championship team, the first African-American quarterback to be named All American First Team QB (1961), and the MVP of the 1962 Rose Bowl.

CHAPTER 8

MOTIVATION AND THE AMERICAN DREAM

I was reminded constantly that making the Run and recovering from probable depression afterward both depended greatly upon my motivation. The question is whether our motivation reflects who we are and what we want from life. If we like and are proud of what we're doing, our actions will be in sync with the positive goals we set. If they are not, we need to re-think our motivation. Most people do what they are motivated to do. If they don't like what they are doing and are not happy they must find out what their real motivation is. Quite often, our desire to criticize others, to hold others in contempt, or to refuse to communicate honestly is a reflection of dissatisfaction we are experiencing in our own lives. We resort to being defensive or stonewalling any question we are asked; ultimately we can even sabotage the projects or goals we ostensibly are pursuing. We set ourselves up for failure, then wonder why we fail. We need to resolve our inner conflicts to enable us to achieve the goals to which we are truly committed. Experts suggest that the best way to stay honest with yourself is to commit your goals to paper. Check back regularly – daily even – to see if your actions support your goals. If not, it's time to reevaluate or rediscover your true motivation.

Most motivation programs note that it is easier to reinforce our goals over the short term than the long term, and thus, many programs outline how we should reassess our goals each night and make to-do lists. The items on the list can be project-oriented or relationally oriented, so that we have achievable goals on a daily basis and are rewarded each day by having leaped over another hurdle. This is what I did. I had a goal for each day, laid out the night before, usually defining the miles to cover and the tasks to accomplish. With the help of my road crew I was able to achieve my daily goals and, more importantly, see that I had achieved them. That helped reinforce my mind and body to continue training the next day, and the next day, and the next...

As the training intensified so did my mental concentration. The pain of my Achilles tendon remained with me but my heart grew each day knowing this Run could help so many families and so many kids. That thought kept the Achilles' tendon pain at bay. I wondered how I could help re-enfranchise this group to the American Dream. The number of single-parent families is staggering — well over thirty-five million at the time of my Run, and growing every day. How can we, as a country and a society, ignore this important group of people to the extent we do? On the one hand, I am convinced we can do much better in supporting and helping single-parent families and their children. On the other hand, I have been greatly astounded at how many people express concern for kids of single-parent families yet don't know what to do about it. What a waste that so many people can feel excluded from participating as whole members of our society, while those not included have no idea how to help. We all have something different and unique to contribute to our communities and to the single-parent families in them. We must focus on the positive, rather than the negative.

In 1968, following the urban riots, the Kerner Commission Report said the United States was heading toward a split into two countries: one black and one white. The report stated that the days of mass immigration were over, so it would now be impossible for blacks to do what earlier immigrants had done—bootstrap up the ladder of social mobility. Instead, the government would have to take care of them. This philosophy wrote off an entire segment of American society. The terrible thing about this report was that it encouraged a "can't-do" rather than "can-do" attitude about big issues, hammering home a destructively negative message.

As it turned out, immigration was anything but over. New immigrants from Asia and Latin America and Eastern Europe kept coming to America. They faced the hardships of changing lands and cultures. They understood the marathon that stood before them if they were to make it. They stood ready to do whatever it took – sacrifice themselves, if necessary, for their children.

There is a pervasive attitude regarding the plight of single-parent families and their children. Americans pay lip service to the need for strong, healthy families, but rarely do we believe this strength and family health can be recovered if, for some reason, it is lost or falters. This disbelief is reflected in government policies that undermine the efforts of families struggling to get on their feet. On a personal level, we ignore or harshly judge the single-parent plight as though these children have nothing to do with us. If one stops to consider it, however, we realize all children have something to do with each of us. At some level, whether through taxes, personal care, or personal relationships, every adult contributes in some way to the raising of every child. Were we not all children once? Despite the negativity surrounding them, single parents and their kids cling to the belief that the American Dream also belongs to them. We cannot afford to write off these families any more than we can afford to write off a whole race or culture.

It seems that so many single parents, so overwhelmed by their every day struggles, come to the same conclusion as the Kerner Report. Single parents believe that, for whatever reason, they just can't make it. Too many feel defeated before they start. They sit down and wait for a hand out or a hand up that never comes. They have lost the personal drive of immigrants who literally make it on their vision and the sweat and toil of their own hands.

Single parents are cultural immigrants, having emigrated from the land of the two-parent family to the land of the single-parent family. Whether they began parenting with a partner or began single parenting by choice, it is a foreign land to live in and a tough choice to have made or had forced upon you.

I am disappointed by the way many business leaders and politicians skirt the issues surrounding single-parent households. Following ideologies and narrow agendas, they ignore the overall good of the community and spend their time raising funds for future campaigns instead of raising awareness of issues of immediate importance – issues such as support for kids of single parents, and for kids in general, or the betterment of immigrants in a land with single parents.

The young people in America receive too many mixed messages. Their vision is lost before it develops. This absence is reflected in their excuses for not being able to make it on their own. Either they feel they do not need help to make it or they feel too needy, believing they must have more help in order to get by. Too often they don't think they have a community behind them, ready to help raise their barns. Kids need the whole community to help them make the right choices and bolster their self-confidence. I hoped my Run would demonstrate that if an old guy like me could make it, so could others – especially the young. I didn't allow doubt to enter my mind. In retrospect, I think that if I hadn't made it in the sense of crossing an official finish line, I would want to be remembered as a man who inspired others to persevere and follow their dreams much as Terry Fox inspired me. I remain in awe of his dedication, his dream, his commitment, and his love for others.

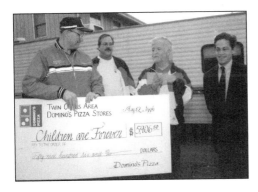

Dominoes Pizza & Sen. Coleman w/check

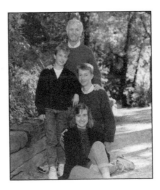

Casual family moment

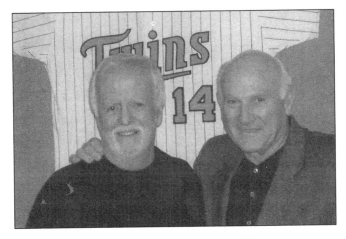

Harmon Killebrew of Minnesota Twins

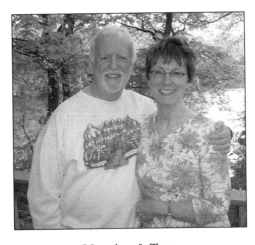

Mary Ann & Terry

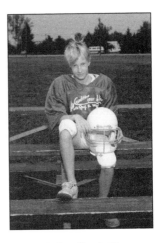

Chris's first football game

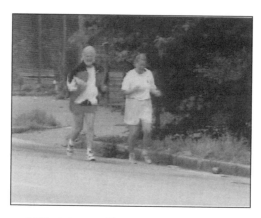

J. Marie joining Terry outside of St. Louis

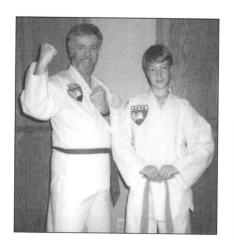

Chris & Terry in Tae Kwan Doe class

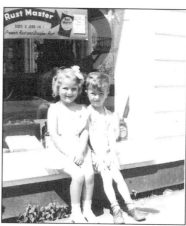

Terry & friend Suzanne as children

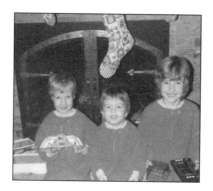

Chris, Jason and Teri Sue

waiting for Santa

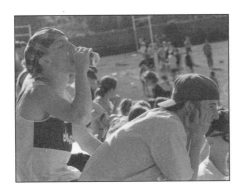

Jason & Chris on track

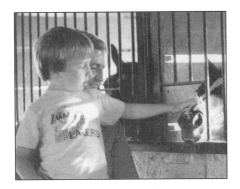

Jason & Terry w/horse

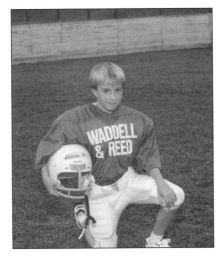

Jason getting ready for game

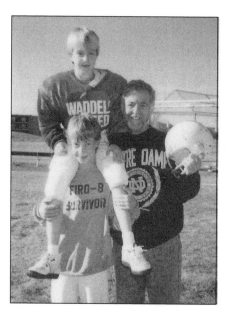

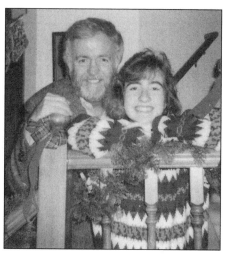

Teri Sue and Terry

Chris & Terry holding up
Jason after football game

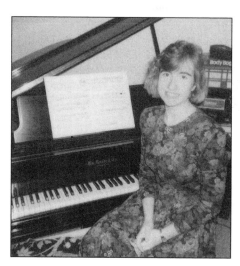

Teri Sue on piano

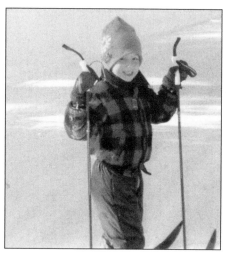

Jason skiing

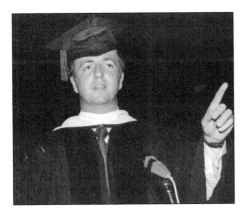

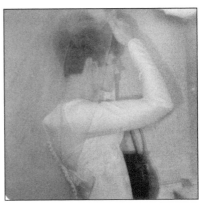

Terry giving college commencement address   Sue preparing for wedding day

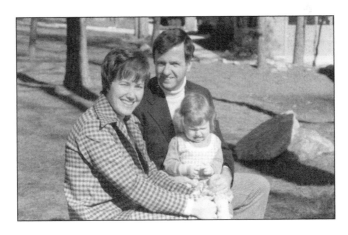

Sue, Terry, and Teri Sue at Atlanta home

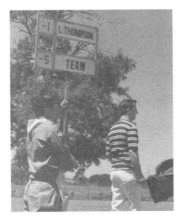

Terry playing in Milwaukee Open Pro Am

"Terry and his son, Chris, need to be highly commended, and also Terry's daughter, Teri Sue, and son, Jason. Their two thousand-mile treks to the 1996 Olympics were truly remarkable. Truly unbelievable. We in America need to say to them, 'We're proud of you.'"

—U.S. Sen. Paul Wellstone of Minnesota, and his wife Sheila Wellstone.

Both died in a plane crash Oct. 25, 2002,
along with their daughter,
three staff members and the two pilots.

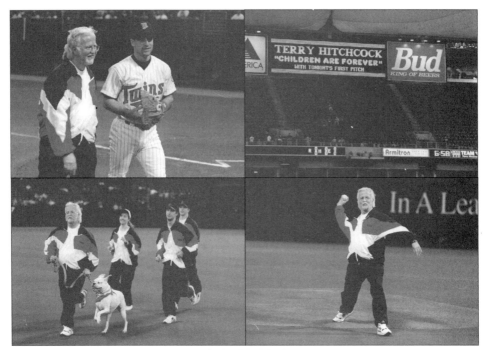

CHAPTER 9

THE SEND-OFF:
WEDNESDAY, MAY 1, 1996

I stood in the center of the Metrodome – the great sports and events stadium at the center of the Twin Cities' urban renewal – surrounded by thousands of cheering fans. The next morning I would wake up early and start my trek of more than two thousand miles to the 1996 Summer Olympics in Atlanta, Georgia. On this night I was on the playing field, meeting some of the Minnesota Twins, throwing out the first pitch, and being serenaded by children as a send-off.

The Metrodome. Home to the Minnesota Twins, who clinched World Series wins in 1987 and 1991. Home to the Minnesota Vikings, four-time participants in the Super Bowl under legendary Head Coach Bud Grant, and a team that was one game away from the Super Bowl twice in the 1990s under their other legendary Head Coach, Dennis Green. It was the first-year home of the Minnesota Timberwolves and site of the 1992 NFL Super Bowl between the Buffalo Bills and the Washington Redskins. And now, on May 1, 1996, at the Minnesota Twins baseball game against Kansas City, it was the place my Run began. The stadium was filled with some of the greatest baseball fans in the world. I know. I have been a Twins fan for many years. Twins fans are wise to the sport and I felt honored to be with them that night.

What a send-off! This was the moment I had waited for; it was exhilarating. It was exciting for everyone who worked directly on the project, and to all who heard our message that day. Imagine being on the field where Kirby Puckett played and Tom Kelly managed. Present that night was Gene Larkin, the hero of game seven of the '91 World Series, and a friend and supporter of mine and of my effort to make a difference. Gene had helped with my spiritual focus during training when it seemed too tough and never-ending. Between him and the thousands in attendance I felt as though I was getting a gigantic group hug.

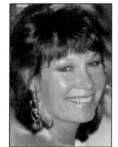

Just prior to the game, as part of the celebration, a dear friend of my family, Bev Asher, presented a poem she had written, *Children Are Forever.* It was a surprise to me, and the crowd at the Metrodome was silent as she read:

If children are forever, and we can lead the way
What is it we need to do to help the children today?
We need to make the difference that starts with love and grows
If children are forever, stand up and let them know.

Children are the future we reach for every day
Their light can only shine so bright if hurting goes away
Our children need the love and hope and best of us each day

The Send-Off: Wednesday, May 1, 1996

If children are forever – giving is the way.
We all can make the difference – let's choose to start today
For once we are a child; that never goes away
Abuse, neglect, the hurt we know can be a yesterday
If children are forever, WE are the way.

Listen to your heart – for it will guide you through
To know that love is what to give and it will make you do
For doing is our hope alive – to make this dream come true
Give your love, give your heart – our children do need you.

Make this day the day we say, I will start anew
Love is what I choose to give, I choose to give to you.
Rise up, let's join together to give the gift of love
To heal the hearts of children, with songs from above.

Next, the Children Are Forever choir sang a song written just for the evening. Their song, *Dreams Come True*, written by their director, Roberta Davis, was later sung many times at fundraisers.

With Teri Sue, Chris, Jason, and Charlie, I ran a lap around the outfield to the applause and cheers of the crowd. Following my short introduction explaining what we were about, the Children Are Forever choir sang the national anthem and pandemonium broke loose. What a crowd! They came to celebrate, to cheer, and to enjoy themselves. After the anthem, I had the thrill of doing what every baseball fan secretly yearns to do, especially those who have played as youngsters: I threw out the first pitch. I used to pitch, dreaming of a pro career, so having the opportunity to throw at the send-off was especially poignant. It wasn't a strike. All I could muster was what I would call a Hitchcock pitch-out. When I received the ball I had pitched I gave it to my good friend Gary Lesley's son, Jake, who accepted it from me with all the joy and enthusiasm of the wide-eyed young boy he was.

Even more wonderful things took place that night. As I left the playing field after throwing out the first pitch I met a number of friends and family. In the group was a little girl who gave me a big hug and handed me her ticket stub. On the stub she had written, "Don't ever give up. Kids depend on you." It was signed, "Dianne Hiatt." What a wonderful thing! It was very special to have her share her feelings, and that night was a special time to receive such a gift. Children can often be our teachers, if we just listen to them. Children reflect what we have taught them. They are us in the looking glass. They see and hear the daily issues of parenting. They are the leaders of tomorrow, but they also unknowingly lead today with their innocence. We need to give them a greater voice.

The governor of Minnesota had issued a proclamation making the following day *Children Are Forever Day*. This was a great recognition for a dream about to come true. I knew that raising awareness of the plight of kids in single-parent families and of every kid's need for a future did not carry an intrinsic, glamorous appeal. My appeal was a practical one: to not throw away our seed corn – the kids – because of circumstances beyond their control or actions taken by others. My goal was to have the MegaMarathon become the event that sparked the beginning of a process for change.

I knew this process must work if we are going to stop skirting and avoiding this issue about children – an issue that affects us all, regardless of whether we are aware of it. This MegaMarathon must draw the gaze and attention of adults so sorely needed by children. I hoped my effort and focus would inspire everyone to never again look away.

The true marvel of the evening was the very special spirit often noted in Upper-Midwesterners. Just think of it. For the Twin Cities to back me, and for a favorite team to give me this kind of time and exposure, showed how compelling my message was. I felt humbled when I realized how credible and trustworthy I was perceived as a man and human being. That trust felt like a wind blowing at my back, pushing me onward toward Atlanta. To me, trust is everything. What happened at that game is what some call synergy. Others call it inspiration. Whatever it was, this great Twin Cities community of the Upper-Midwest was inspired and they, in turn, returned lasting inspiration to me. They were energized and gave energy back to me, energy that fueled me, enabling me to complete this difficult and daring feat.

The *Children Are Forever* foundation sold T-shirts and hats at the game. Many of the fans visited with us and wished us a safe trip as we began to mentally prepare for the next morning, when I would leave the warmth and comfort of my home and begin traveling the two thousand miles to Atlanta.

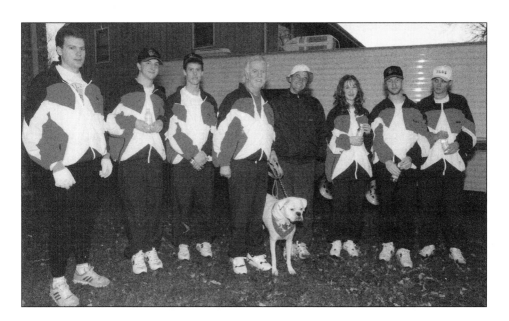

Day 1
Route: Battle Creek area of St. Paul, through Hastings, to Miesville, Minn.
Weather: Cloudy and cool, with some rain
Comment: Excitement followed by terrible pain all over my body after completing first
day. I wonder if I will survive the first week.

DAY 1: THURSDAY, MAY 2.

I awoke at 4:30 a.m. and had a moment's pause as I pondered the fact that, though I had a map, I was in many ways heading off into the unknown. My mind raced along a dark roadway before I took a single stride, then my training took over. I might have been apprehensive but I was ready.

My road crew gathered and packed the thirty-two-foot trailer and one-ton truck that we had picked up the previous night. My dog Charlie would run with me a few miles each day, while Chris and Jason coordinated the advance team. The team was composed of several other young adults, ages seventeen to nineteen, all from single-parent families. The plan called for them to handle all logistics of the Run. They would carry all our supplies and food in the trailer, truck, and two cars.

By 6:00 a.m. a crowd of friends, bundled against the morning cold, had gathered outside my home to wish me success and provide the hugs I needed as I ventured south. Many friends and supporters were there, including such special people as John Williams of WCCO, Dr. Roth, J. Marie Fieger, John Pope, Perry Williams, Greg Dittrich, Rick Marklund, Larry Kline and Zak Manuszak. They had come to run the first mile with me and provide encouragement for my first day on the highway. Norm Coleman, then mayor of St. Paul, was also present. He

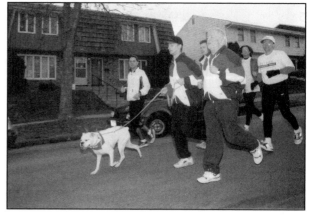

shook my hand and shared his support for parents everywhere, particularly the single parents who struggle each day with their own parenting marathons. He proclaimed May 2, 1996, "Terry Hitchcock and Children Are Forever Day," and read his proclamation to everyone present. The media were on hand to share in this special moment – various television, newspaper, and radio people waited outside as I reviewed our checklist. Most of my neighbors stood outside and waved, many with banners and signs, delivering their support. The banner we broke at the start said, "Good Luck Terry & *Children Are Forever* From Your Friends at Petters Warehouse Direct." Tom Petters had supported us in many ways.

The banner dropped and we were off. Charlie bolted ahead, pulling at his leash. All that we had planned for during the past seventeen months had begun. The Run had started. I experienced a surge of excitement and adrenaline as we took off. Some friends ran with us for one block. Others ran for the first mile. Then it was just me, Scott Meier, and Charlie. When Charlie became winded we returned him to the trailer, but Scott stayed with me for the first twenty-three miles. I persevered for another eight, for a total of thirty-one miles on the first day.

As I ran, all I could think was, what a glorious Thursday morning. It had finally arrived, the first day of our event, MegaMarathon '96. In my mind, as we ran, I replayed the interviews I had at various TV and radio stations around the Twin Cities. WCCO-AM KFAN-AM, KDWB-FM, KWWK-FM, WBOB-AM, AAHS, KSTP-AM, WCCO-TV, KARE-TV, KSTP-TV, KMSPTV, WFTC-TV, KLGT-TV – they had all contributed to the much-needed exposure for the Run. I reviewed in my mind the wonderful stories and coverage we received in our two great hometown newspapers, the *Minneapolis Star-Tribune* and the *St. Paul Pioneer Press*. I also recalled the coverage from other fine publications: the *Winona Daily*, *EastSide Review*, *Bloomington Sun-Current*, *Minnesota Parent*, *Young Adult Press*, *Lifestyle Choices*, and *Northwest Health Club Magazine*. By bringing our story to their respective audiences, each of these publications had helped spread the word and contribute to the success of the Run.

I felt as though I was running on air. I was so excited to be able to finally live this wonderful moment – a dream come true. I wish every man and woman could someday share in this special feeling. As I ran on this first day, it occurred to me that the many others who helped make this exciting endeavor possible were all bound together by the same dream. We all have dreams; often a given individual is the sole believer in his or her personal dream. And now, here I was, not only seeing my dream come true but being sustained by the reality that the citizens of these two great cities also believed in this dream and supported it.

My mind floated between the trivial and the wondrous as I ran. I wondered how else I could invite others to share in this special dream-fulfillment feeling. The reaction at the Metrodome send-off had demonstrated that many others share the dream of calling attention to the predicament of kids in single-parent families and recognize its importance. *Dreams are so infectious* – I thought, *if*

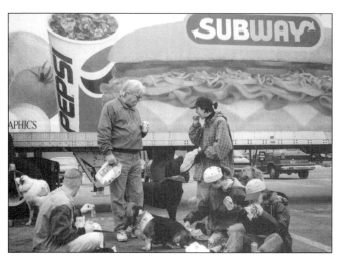

this Run can help fuel the dreams of the many millions of single parents and their children in this country, then the pain and agony of the training and the Run will be well worth it. I hoped I could inspire them not only to continue to keep their chins up as they ran their daily marathons, but also to take steps to help improve their situations. I just knew we could make a difference – I knew that we already had. We already had a Boot Hockey tournament in St. Paul, a Woof Woof Walk, meetings with Child Care Aware Groups, we had been adopted by the Diamond Path Elementary School in Apple Valley, and soon would host a Mother's Day and Father's Day celebration at Knott's Camp Snoopy in the Mall of America. How could we not do some good?

Many more fundraisers were to take place during the Run, planned in order to pay for everything. This was more than an event – it was I hoped the beginning of a wonderful grassroots movement. With such support, I certainly felt I could last the ten and a half weeks of the Run. I knew it would be hot and dangerous, not only to my health and body, but dangerous being on the road and facing the traffic and crazy drivers.

A children's radio station, AAHS Radio, which broadcast to major cities around the country, had asked me to come to their studio before my appearance at the Metrodome and talk with kids who called in from all over the country. During the afternoon, kids called from Seattle, Denver, New York, and Memphis. They asked questions and shared their support for what kids go through each day. It was gratifying to hear the various stories and I knew that the focus of *Children Are Forever* was right on target. As a single parent I knew in my heart that my purpose in this particular part of my life was to somehow make a difference for kids. I knew that God had set aside this time for me to make that difference. I just knew that He was allowing me to make this two thousand-mile trek to Atlanta to honor single-parent families and their children. I felt He also wanted this Run to be a spiritual journey for me, personally. As Terry Fox said, "I guess by believing in God you can't lose."

I had also spent time with radio host John Williams of WCCO the day before the send-off. I first met with John weeks before. He questioned my sanity. He had just finished running the Boston Marathon, was terribly sore, and walked funny as we discussed my plans. John knew I was serious, but of course he was remembering his own pain after a single marathon. He held an incredulous smile as I explained my plans to each day run and finish at least one twenty-six-mile marathon – seventy-five marathons in as many days. Impossible, John's eyes seemed to say as we sat across from each other in the WCCO newsroom. But by then, impossible was not a word in my vocabulary. I had already run many personal and professional marathons. This would, in some ways, be the easiest as it had a specific path, a specific time frame, and most important, a specific moment when it would end. I didn't mind John's reaction. I was amused. After all, doctors and experienced runners all over said it was impossible, that no one could do it, that the Run would kill me. But I knew the secret of Sir Edmund Hillary and Roger Bannister – someone is always going to be the first at what is currently thought impossible. So why not be the first to do this?

Seventy-five marathons in seventy-five consecutive days meant covering the distance at a steady pace, not a rapid one. The plan was not to run a championship race of two to three hours, but to take four to six hours, depending upon the condition of the terrain, the weather, and my feet and legs. I had to pace myself. The only opponent was attitude, and I had the right attitude to make it. At that first meeting I could see John was unconvinced, but I didn't mind. I wasn't letting the birds nest in my hair, and I knew the best way to change the skeptics' minds was to show them the impossible was anything but.

After thirty-one miles we stopped for the day. Thirty-one miles! The first of seventy-five marathons (and then some) was now history. That first night, we parked the trailer in the parking lot of the Miesville Mud Hens baseball team in southern Minnesota. The caravan was in place. All the necessary roles were filled with willing, eager volunteers. My mind was in glorious wonderment, but not my body; it was already sore. The level of pain began to build as the night wore on. Several friends came down from the Twin Cities to celebrate the first night, and at first, I enjoyed their company. They made it possible. We would succeed.

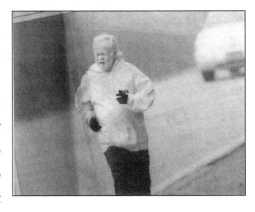

Then, my body quit cooperating and I wasn't able to enjoy their presence any longer. I stayed up as long as I could, until I was too weary and uncomfortable. Nice as it was to see everyone, my body was already crying out for no more. I began to wonder what I was doing to myself, and whether I could really last the first week or even a few more days, let alone two and a half months. Was it worth the excitement? Could I pay the daily price of admission – the pain and discomfort – for seventy-five days?

This was certainly not like the training I had endured for the last seventeen months. Yes, halfway through my training I had a heart attack. And yes, it was frightening. But this was somehow different. I had never run so far in a given day. My feet hurt, my back hurt, everything hurt. God only knew how I was going to last the full duration, so that's where I put my faith. He never gives you more than you can bear. Perhaps I would become more accustomed to the pain. I was told my body could adapt, so I fell asleep counseling myself to give it time. Be patient.

Day 2
Route: Miesville, through Cannon Falls and Hader, to Zumbrota, Minn.
Weather: Cold, with a hard rain
Comment: Working through the pain, and trying to understand what my body will need. Bananas are becoming quick friends.

DAY 2: FRIDAY, MAY 3

On the second day I completed another thirty miles, making it to Zumbrota, Minnesota. The day went smoothly and the team members did their jobs with no real problems. My body continued to react to the beating it was taking. My feet were sore, my heels and calves were on the verge of cramping every hour or so. So far, I had not eaten as many bananas as my nutrition program called for. I knew I needed to take in as much potassium as possible, but I was already sick of bananas. Thank goodness it wasn't very hot. On the other hand, the cold and rainy weather wasn't much better. The dampness seemed to spread the soreness throughout my body.

I dreaded the pain of leg cramps during the past year and a half while I trained. I felt I could deal with other types of pain, but I found it scary to wake up in the middle of the night with my calves in knots, having to spend precious sleep time kneading the cramps out. I wished for a physical therapist or masseurs to bring along; that would have been wonderful. I wondered how I would deal with knots every night on my way to Atlanta. I had better break down and eat more bananas.

Day 3
Route: Zumbrota, through Pine Island, Oronoco and Douglas, to Rochester, Minn.
Weather: Cold and wet, again. Dampness goes right through me.
    Comment: Celebration in Rochester. People's smiling faces keep us going.

DAY 3: THURSDAY, MAY 4

We headed toward Rochester, Minnesota on Day 3. I secretly wished for the Mayo Clinic to be waiting with open arms to relieve my soreness. I had to settle for the Mayor of Rochester's proclamation of *Children Are Forever Day*. That provided a little relief for my sore feet. Little did I know it was just the start of a long, but very happy day.

I felt fortunate and grateful to have my family as part of the team. My older son, Chris, was in charge of my eating schedule and keeping me hydrated. He provided water bottles every twenty minutes. Sometimes I carried the bottle in my hand and drank as I ran, or sometimes I stopped to drink, then continued on my way. Either way, hydration was a critical factor, and it meant the world to me to have Chris taking on that responsibility. Jason kept up with our supplies, taking care of both my needs and those of the rest of the team. Teri Sue remained in the Twin Cities with J. Marie Fieger and Perry Williams, helping with fundraising, mailings, telephone calls and faxes.

As I mentioned earlier, the remaining road team was composed of kids from single-parent families. Kim, looking for professional experience, signed on to handle PR and finances on the road. Mike and Andy were general troubleshooters. They were all volunteers and all welcome, but all young, just out of school with little experience handling 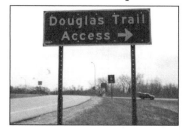 some of the tough issues that came up, it seemed, every day. They wanted to take frequent breaks and couldn't understand why I did not.

Still, on the third day we completed an unbelievable forty miles. We spent most of the day on the Douglas Trail, a beautiful running, skating, and bike path from Zumbrota to Rochester. We finished our day in Rochester at a Tires Plus, meeting with new and old friends, selling our T-shirts, and eating pizza provided by a local Domino's Pizza. Pizza wasn't exactly on the menu for me, but I ate a piece anyway.

I also received a complimentary massage from Gary Dix of Rochester. Gary and his wife invited us to their home, where we used the hot tub located outside in a beautiful, scenic portion of their land. Deer and other animals roamed nearby. The massage and the hot tub were really appreciated. I slept with little pain or discomfort that night.

With so much solitary time on the road, it was easy to dwell on the overwhelming number of days and miles ahead. However, our family of sponsors continued to support us as we wove through the daily obstacles. Perkins Restaurant was great, and helped me look forward to the dinners, hospitality, and graciousness in the coming days. The sponsors truly were our best friends. I knew they were motivated by promotional exposure, but I was sure they also believed in the Run and our cause. They served us well and provided an oasis whenever we were overcome by the immensity of the project. Just like individual volunteers, the sponsors were crucial to our success.

Day 4
Route: Rochester, through Dover, to near St. Charles, Minn.
Weather: Cold, lots of rain. Wind pelts my face while running.
Comment: Wind pelted my face all day. I changed clothes and shoes six times, between dodging cars, to keep dry.

DAY 4: THURSDAY, MAY 5

On Sunday morning we left Rochester and headed southeast toward St. Charles, Minnesota. It rained much of the day and cold wind battered my face. I had to keep changing clothes, even with a double layer of rain gear. The day seemed especially long; the rain hit me in the face with real force and stung as it pelted my body. The cars that day seemed less polite than before. The road narrowed and vehicles competed with Charlie and me for the pavement. We had to jump out of the way of oncoming traffic several times. I was getting pretty good at the dodging game but I didn't like putting Charlie at risk. Maybe, I thought, the Vikings and Coach Green needed a good running back for the upcoming year – or maybe not. If only there was a dodge ball league for guys in their fifties.

We camped that night at the Lazy D campground outside St. Charles. The team played baseball and touch football, and cooked marshmallows over a campfire. For the first time in what seemed like an eternity my body allowed me to be sort of whole again – with the emphasis on "sort of." The pains and aches were less intense. I thought I might get through the first week after all.

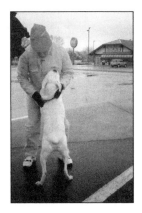

Friends from Minneapolis drove down to be with us and helped prepare a great Italian dinner. The team members and I put banners on our trailer and I took a shower for the first time in four days. Unfortunately, the trailer had no heat, no hot water, and no electricity. In fact, none of these things had functioned properly since the beginning of the Run. The kids hadn't been able to resolve the problems and the nights were still very cold. Our ability to cook hot meals was limited, too. There is only so much a group of city-dwellers can do over a campfire. Still, I fell asleep thinking that tomorrow was a new day and I had just over twenty-six miles to cover. I also realized that I would not be running straight south at all; roads under repair, detours, and other situations meant I would zigzag all the way to Atlanta. It was a straight line to Atlanta on the map but it was already obvious that my route would wind all the way.

Day 5
Route: St. Charles, through Lewiston and Stockton, to Winona, Minn.
Weather: Gray skies, brief rains and lots of wind
   Comment: Talked with large college crowd. Pain is terrible and distracting.

DAY 5: THURSDAY, MAY 6

On Day 5 we traveled to Winona, Minnesota, where I was scheduled to speak at Winona State University. I also met with representatives of the Watkins Company. We enjoyed Watkins, an old and stable corporation known for spices, seasonings, and home care products marketed throughout the United States, Canada, and New Zealand. They gave us a few gifts and their best wishes, and then a Winona Press newspaper reporter interviewed me while I jogged on the highway near town. He wrote a wonderful, inspirational article, including a front-page action photo of me running. Winona is a beautiful town with a colorful history – I'm so glad its people support those like me who try to create change for some special good.

While the team moved on, Kim's car had to be towed back to the Twin Cities. Her brakes gave out and were no longer safe for driving. We decided to have Chris's car brought out from home to replace Kim's. We also found two defective batteries in the trailer. I knew this kind of thing could happen on ventures such as ours, but each issue we faced was compounded for me by the daily pounding on my body and the emotional stress. Any issue was potentially overwhelming and I forced myself to keep my eyes straight ahead. I couldn't concentrate on those issues – my focus needed to be on the hourly rhythm of putting one foot in front of the other. There were many moments when I wanted to quit; all my training couldn't prepare me for how painful, lonely, and difficult the actual Run turned out to be.

Day 6
Route: Winona to near La Crosse, Wis.
Weather: Windy, cloudy and cold. Brief rains
Comment: Friends joined us to celebrate. Pain still is prevalent, but my body begins to accept its fate. Kid's laughing faces keep us going.

DAY 6: THURSDAY, MAY 7

As I ran across the Minnesota-Wisconsin bridge into La Crosse, Wisconsin, something happened that pulled me out of the funk I had been in. As we entered Wisconsin, my son Chris leaned out the car window and shouted that we only had six states to go. He recommended I get a horse, then laughed and offered to just drive me the rest of the way.

The hearty impetuousness of his youth snapped me right out of my mini-depression. I realized that I was six and two-thirds percent of the way to Atlanta. (Amazing what the mind does to alleviate boredom as the body methodically plods along.) I began thinking anew that this could really work; we could pull it off. My determination surged back, and suddenly I returned to a positive state of mind.

The La Crosse Tribune followed Charlie and me along the highway and into La Crosse. They interviewed me and took photos for a front-page article the next day. The local television and radio stations followed and interviewed me and the team. Upon arriving in La Crosse, we met once again at a Tires 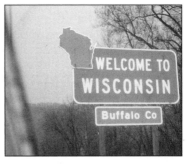 Plus to regroup and celebrate. Perry Williams, J. Marie Fieger, and Michael Durant joined us there and helped the road team members with the press and public relations.

Both Perry and J. Marie asked how I was doing. I said I felt wonderful. In truth, the pain was excruciating. But seeing them there changed everything for me once again. I marveled at how the mind can short-circuit the pain of the body, especially with nothing more than the sight of a friendly face or a warm smile. They asked what I looked forward to. I answered that I just hoped it wouldn't rain on Day 7. Perry and J. Marie wondered how I would make it the rest of the way and I responded by saying, "I think if you can find one thing you really believe in to hold onto, you can do anything."

We had mounted a billboard on the side of the trailer and encouraged local kids to cover it with their handprints. The kids were great; it seemed like half of La Crosse showed up for that one evening. By the time we went to bed the billboard was covered with small handprints and scrawled names. Being part of the Run obviously made a world of difference to each child. It made them feel a part of something significant and their happiness sparked my own.

Day 7 and 8
Route: La Crosse, through Stoddard and Genoa, to DeSoto, Wis.
Weather: Rain, Rain (Go away!)
   Comment: I miss my friends and tired of the cold and dampness.

DAYS 7 & 8: WEDNESDAY & THURSDAY, MAY 8-9

The team, Charlie and I continued to push further into Wisconsin. My path followed the Mississippi River as it wound around the countryside. The scenery was breathtaking and I stopped many times to watch an eagle catch a piece of wind and soar into the highways of the sky. It was a beautiful sight. Back on my own highway the road seemed narrower and trucks and cars more often pushed Charlie and me off the road. As yet, I didn't view this challenge as too dangerous.

I saw a lot of wildlife as I ran. Herds of deer were everywhere and Chris had an exciting experience while waiting for me on the shoulder of the highway. He came across a fawn trying to follow its mother over a wooden fence – the doe had jumped the fence and was waiting for the fawn on the other side. Chris saw that the fawn was unable to jump the fence or crawl under. He went over and calmed the fawn, then helped it maneuver the fence to join its mother. Chris felt great, and it was wonderful to see his expression of pleasure as he watched the fawn run with its mother into the woods.

As we continued on, a thousand thoughts raced through my head. Every day of the Run so far the weather had been dismally unfriendly. Each day it had rained with a cold, damp wind. Although I continued to change my clothes every few hours, the dampness entered every part of my being.

Water was weighing me down like an anvil on my back. Being burdened by water is a terrible thing for a runner. Ideally, you strive to feel light on your feet, as if your body is but a feather floating down the road. Water was the enemy, sapping my will along with my energy. I was soaked when I completed each of those first days, and by halfway through the second week we had to wash at least two-dozen changes of clothing. I fell asleep each night praying that the sun would soon shine and warmer weather would prevail. I didn't want to quit, but I felt I might be forced to if the weather didn't improve.

I already missed my friends and their hugs. I needed lots of physical reassurance. Loneliness set in again. I felt no one could understand my situation without experiencing it firsthand. I didn't always understand it myself, and in that confusion a hug meant more than ever before.

Cold and dampness produced a unique type of pain. Even bundled in warm, loose clothes in my sleeping bag I shivered all night and woke up constantly. I contended with not only the pain of steady running and the abuse on my body, but also with a chill that permeated every part of my being. It had to stop, I told myself. I wasn't prepared for this. It was like signing up with a recruiter who promised Hawaii and sent you to Alaska. Only in this case, I was both the recruiter and the recruit.

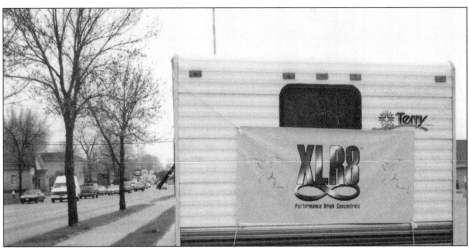

Day 9
Route: DeSoto, through Mount Sterling, to Seneca, Wis.
Weather: More rain!
    Comment: Quiet and lonely. The team begins to question its commitment.

DAY 9: FRIDAY, MAY 10

In the morning Andy and the guys loaded the trailer and prepared for the day's drive. I took off running. After a while they caught up and asked how I was doing. I offered my latest mantra: "I've felt better." It had been a long three miles and it was just the start. If possible, the rain seemed wetter than I had ever experienced. And cold. I couldn't stop shivering, even while running.

As I ran I worried about our group. The trailer still had power problems; it was almost impossible to cook. We were getting little, if any, heat. Andy was doing his best. He gave daily briefings to the crew on what to expect on the road the next day, but they didn't seem to be really trying to deal with the hardships. I tried to be encouraging and to lead by example, but it was a hard example to set when I felt so physically and mentally drained. Even talking felt like a waste of precious energy.

Day 10
Route: Seneca, through Eastman, to Wauzeka, Wis.
Weather: Cold and windy, yet again
Comment: Met some campers. The cold and dampness continues to wear at my resolve.

DAY 10: SATURDAY, MAY 11

I met with a number of groups who wanted to know more about the Children Are Forever Foundation, a National Heritage Foundation. Every day of the Run, numerous people came up to one or more of us and introduced themselves. Kids wanted to touch Charlie and talk to him. I found it fun and heartwarming to talk with all the kids we met. On the highway, cars and trucks honked and drivers waved when they saw our caravan, with Charlie and me running a short distance in front of the trailer and cars.

I was trying to run as much as possible, but when my knees hurt I walked a short distance, then resumed running when they felt better. Switching from running to walking helped, but it also slowed me down. I almost preferred to put up with the knee pain to get the day's running done as soon as possible, just to get out of the elements. A trailer with no heat was still better than no protection at all. It's amazing what you come to consider luxurious in a time when no luxuries are at hand.

On this Saturday, a group of campers asked us to join them for a cookout. It was fun, and we had the first good food in what seemed like a long time, though it had really only been a little more than a week. The campers had come from several states and we joined their annual get-together. Most of the families had known one another for years – it struck me what a wonderful tradition this was for their kids to experience. We shared stories of the Run to date, as well as how neglected single-parent families were in general. Everyone was supportive of what we were doing and they promised to take our story to their communities. The cookout was the epitome of what the Run was all about—families. Traditions such as this are wonderful, especially when they include kids of single-parent families. The kids connected to a wider range of other significant adults, becoming part of something bigger than themselves.

"Although I did not physically accompany Terry as he ran his marathons, I would like to invite others to join me in becoming lifelong partners with Terry in his endless journey – that of ensuring a solid future for children everywhere."

—Fred Hoiberg

Former NBA player and Assistant General Manager
for the Minnesota Timberwolves

CHAPTER 10

DAYS 11 THROUGH 20

Day 11
Route: Wauzeka to Prairie du Chien, Wis.
Weather: Plenty of gray sky.
   Comment: Few towns and fewer people. My son, Jason, returned home

DAY 11: SUNDAY, MAY 12.

Very few towns waited in our path on this day. To break up the monotony, Andy took PR photos of me and members of the support team wearing products from our sponsors, including RUDS, Breathe Right, Polar Heart Monitor, Head Lites, Roller Blades, Bennett's Cycle, Perkins, Wigwam Socks, Natural Ovens, XLR8, AT&T, West Link, Gargoyles, and others.

My son Jason flew back to the Twin Cities to resume high school studies set to begin on May 13. It was wonderful that his school let him have two weeks off to be with the team. I couldn't picture starting the Run without him. He planned to continue working with J. Marie, Perry, and the rest of the Minneapolis support team. While on the road, he was responsible for our supply inventory; it was a difficult job and he'd done well at it, including setting up a system to make the task easier for the others. Still, his return home was sad and difficult for me. I knew I would miss him, but education comes first. It was easier for Chris, who had decided not to return to college this semester. High school just didn't work that way.

I began to realize, ever so slowly, that the loss of even one team member made the group feel much smaller. I hoped we wouldn't have any more attrition; what would we do without everyone handling his or her job? Andy was covering the advance detail. He sought out the media in the field and worked with J. Marie and Perry back home to set up events as I came into each town or city. Mike and Kim had to relocate our vehicles each day. The trailer was over 32-feet long and we had to find a home for it every night. State campgrounds were prime real estate for our caravan, but they weren't always available. Mike and Kim worked hard to make sure I was as comfortable as possible. And Chris – Chris kept me alive. He spent his days providing me with proper nutrition and watching out for my health and safety. He was on top of how I was feeling at every moment. He provided me with liquid every twenty minutes. It was a tough and demanding job. All their jobs were tough and demanding and everyday I was grateful for their generosity.

Day 12
Route: Prairie du Chien to south of Garnavillo, Iowa.
Weather: Sunshine, just a bit
Comment: People begin to meet us on the highways. We received hugs from families. My body still struggles with each step. The rain suits and traffic get me at times.

DAY 12: MONDAY, MAY 13

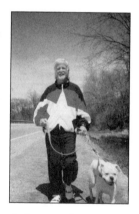

The first day of true sunshine arrived as we entered Iowa. Just a little, mind you, but real, bona fide sunlight. I was scheduled to run more than twenty-nine miles that day, and the change of weather felt great. I eagerly slathered on the sun block, but Old Sol merely teased, letting us know he was up there before abandoning us to the clouds. Still, that brief warmth did much to rekindle my motivation.

An even greater motivator waited at the side of the road as I ran through a residential area. A little boy and his family stood at the end of their driveway. When I stopped, the boy asked if I was the man running to Atlanta. His name was Johnny and his dad said they had been at the Twins game on May 1. Johnny wanted to give me a hug and a great gift: a ticket stub from the game. On the ticket were the signatures of Johnny and his three best friends. Above the names was written, "We love you. Don't get hurt."

This was exactly the kind of thing that kept me going – imagine, waiting on the side of the road for me to arrive, and making certain I knew how he felt. Thanks Johnny, and thanks Shirley, Bill, and Chuck.

We still had no heat, hot water, or electricity in our trailer. Mike and Andy planned to take the trailer to a dealer the next day to see if it could be fixed. Also we had not been able to repair a broken window and door lock on our truck. I knew these were issues we needed to overcome. Still, mundane nuisances created a lot of difficulty as we tried to make the MegaMarathon happen. I found it very hard, even impossible, to concentrate on what I had ahead of me when problems arose and changed my focus. Worse, not having heat made us long for our warm beds at home.

I was still having difficulty with the dampness my body couldn't seem to shake. I shivered throughout each night and couldn't even alleviate the chill with a warm shower. Every day these little things seemed like great reasons to call it quits and go back. But I couldn't. Why? I wasn't sure. Stubbornness? Pride? Unwillingness to admit defeat? Fear of returning home and facing everyone as a failure? Of course, it was all these things. Although I had always used those attributes as daily motivators, I relied mainly on my Vermont ethic. When my sense of purpose flagged I thought of the kids and what raising awareness of them could mean. My legs said, *no, stop*. My heart said, *yes, continue*. My mind said, *I will*, and my heart and mind won.

The team was also feeling the hardship. I hated thinking pessimistically, but I wouldn't have been surprised to hear that the whole team wanted to or would return home before the trek was actually over. I didn't know what I'd do if that happened, but I firmly believed God was with me and would carry me if necessary. In fact, He must have already carried me many times so far, because I had no human explanation for how I had been able to continue. He surely does work miracles, and I was thankful for my own faith. There was a time earlier in my life when I would have just packed everything up and gone home. But now, at age 57, I saw the world a little differently and knew that somehow I would be able to make it to Atlanta.

I didn't know how I had done it, and I could hardly believe I had come this far. I attributed some of my early success to the wonderful love and support from my many supporters and sponsors back home. These gifts from God kept me going mile after mile. Perry, Greg, Rick, Larry, and J. Marie, in particular, kept the daily cheering going and were a real help to me. They and others had done much for the cause. I particularly didn't want to disappoint them. Thinking about them helped me make the next step, and the next mile, and the next day.

By this time, Charlie and I had run well over three-hundred miles. I averaged more than thirty-one miles per day, with Charlie by my side a few miles a day. He was my other motivator and trainer. I had to be careful not to overextend myself, a rather ironic concern in light of the overall project. The extended weather forecast showed continued rain and cold weather, so this day's sun was probably just a hint at what was to come some ways off. I could hardly wait for warmer weather; too hot would be more to my liking than too cold. The rain suits were bulky and made it difficult to be flexible when traffic was heavy and close to me. Once again, it was amazing what I had come to consider a luxury – I was looking forward to the day I could run without sweatshirts and pants.

Day 13
Route: Garnavillo, through Guttenburg, to Luxenburg, Iowa.
Weather: Cloudy, slight wind
Comment: Quiet day. A few close calls with trucks and drivers out to get a jogger. The run is turning into more of a mental than a physical exercise.

DAY 13: TUESDAY, MAY 14

In Guttenberg, Iowa, I experienced another unique act of kindness. A mailman drove behind me, blinking his yellow lights so I could run down a very long and dangerous hill with the protection of his Jeep. Two weeks earlier, a large trailer truck had turned over descending this same hill and the driver was seriously injured. Running down it would have put my life in serious jeopardy. I had already known plenty of scares on some of the highways. In my macabre moments, I joked that I should start an Olympic event for traffic dodging. I don't know if I could have made that hill without the mailman's assistance. He was just one example of many people coming to my aid seemingly from nowhere. Thanks to them, I remained in one piece and was able to move forward. The dangers were real, but so was the generosity. I told myself that as long as my body kept responding, I would happily accept more of both.

Day 14
Route: Luxemburg to Dubuque, Iowa.
Weather: Warming up. Heavy clouds but no rain!
    Comment: Lots of interviews. Kids follow us all over. The team is getting restless.

DAY 14: WEDNESDAY, MAY 15

The Run brought me to Dubuque, Iowa. Once again, the media was great. KATF-FM and KDTH-AM interviewed me for their morning shows. KDUB interviewed the team. *The Telegraph Herald* talked with us and did a great story on single-parent families. *The Gazette*, KWWL-TV, and KCRG-TV, all from Cedar Rapids, were present as well.

The long run on Day 14 left both Charlie and me in some pain as we arrived at Toys R Us, which had agreed to provide us with space and an opportunity to sell our T-shirts and hats. Throughout the time that Charlie was on the road with me, I watched him very closely to make certain he was all right and his excitement of running with me did not overtake his well being. When not running with me, Charlie would ride in the car with Chris and help scout the condition of the highways ahead. About every three miles

Chris would hand me something to eat and drink, and on occasion give me a fresh ice pack. That day I found a large group of people waiting and cheering us on, so I turned off the message of pain in my body. Perry Williams joined the team for the afternoon and evening, providing vital support with his hugs and positive attitude. More kids added their handprints to our billboard. It was fun watching them write their names and leave messages for the kids further down the road.

It was a wonderful day, but still, I was sad. I really missed Jason. He was a good leader, and a great son. His absence grew even more poignant as problems developed on the crew. The kids began arguing more frequently. Mike and Andy seemed to have endless discussions about the trailer batteries, but the problem still wasn't resolved. The bickering and indecision wore me out, but I knew they were young and that I had asked a lot of them.

I wasn't surprised when Andy approached me to discuss his sense of things. He told me he felt he could serve everyone better by working back home; he wanted to return to the Twin Cities. I told myself this could be for the best; the kids had all signed on as equals, each with a role, but Andy wanted more independent authority. People work best when their skills fit the situation and their gifts can best be utilized. The road might not have been the best fit for Andy, so we agreed he should go back and work with Perry and J. Marie. Perry could certainly use all the dedicated help he could get, and Andy could provide much-needed support with faxing and maintaining forward contacts for the road team as we continued southward. I knew he would do great work back in the Twin Cities.

I was down to a support crew of three – make that four, counting Charlie. I told myself we could adapt; we could adjust. We integrated Andy's work into the others', just as we had when Jason left. After all, the ability to adapt is a hallmark trait of creatures with opposable thumbs. I was feeling a little let down from the new departure.

I learned a powerful lesson from this small crisis. I had signed on kids all from single-parent families, believing they would have a special sense of the mission and be able to do more, take on more. But I was guilty of stereotyping and ignoring the importance of experience. They may have a better understanding of the problems and pains of being kids of single parents, but that by itself doesn't instill the motivation and desire to work hard on a mission such as the MegaMarathon. Even if their special insight does motivate them, I needed to remember that they were still kids, with kids' level of maturity. Ironically, I had them again performing the roles of missing adults. The fact that they came from single-parent families, instead of increasing their sympathy and motivation, could just as easily cause stress and overwhelm them beyond their tolerance. Had I been fair?

Day 15
Route: Dubuque to Cascade, Iowa.
Weather: Rain and lightening
 Comment: Nothing exciting, but Chris begins to appreciate the Run and its purpose.

DAY 15: THURSDAY, MAY 16

A wonderful and remarkable thing happened Thursday, a moment I'll never forget. My son Chris asked a little girl why she thought his dad was doing all this running. She stood there and pondered the question, looked at me, turned to Chris, looked him straight in the eye and said, "Because we are fragile." Her voice was sure and without hesitation. My son looked at me and winked; I looked at him, and we knew that somehow we had to get to Atlanta.

She was right. This sweet little girl already knew life, the importance of our mission, and that this world must protect its fragile and innocent – its children. As our children are our most important resource, the future of our country, we need to protect and develop that resource. That goes for all parents, single or not. Single parents often need an extra bit of support, but we all need to learn how to care for our fragile futures.

Day 16
Route: Cascade, through Monticello, to Anamosa, Iowa.
Weather: Less wind and rain
Comment: I spoke in front of elementary classes and adult audiences. The kids understand when you tell them you are doing it for them.

DAY 16: FRIDAY, MAY 17

The past two days took me through Cascade and Anamosa, Iowa, covering more than 56 miles. Most of the countryside was farmland and provided little distraction, so I began talking to the cows and horses along the way. Running along a relatively deserted road caused me to dream, make wishes, and talk to anything that moved. I couldn't help myself. Country roads accentuated the loneliness of running, and the cows and horses were an attentive audience.

They listened well and never talked back. Besides, I had things to say, and I was already accustomed to talking with Charlie. Somehow, my one-sided conversations with him felt far more productive than simply talking to myself. The media picked up on this new habit and probably would have questioned my new quirk, but then again, talking to horses was hardly quirkier than running two thousand miles.

The billboard with children's handprints and our Children Are Forever sign announced our presence at yet another campground. More and more people were recognizing my face and the story as we stopped in towns across the heartland. A few days earlier, I made a statement that if kids are our future we need a Secretary of Children. I wished I could share my thoughts with the President of the United States.

On May 17 I met with the students, teachers, and principal of Grant Woods Elementary School. It was always delightful to meet with school groups and experience their reactions as I explained why I was making the Run. They were eager, excited, and full of questions. The most frequently asked questions were how long would it take to get there, and why was I doing it.

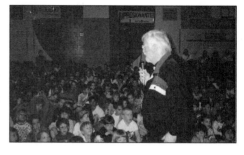

Kids seemed to glow when they heard that this effort was for them.

I believe that more often we need to let our children know we do things for them, that we are concerned about them, and that we love them. Kids are acutely attuned to the false ring of the sanctimonious declaration that something is for their own good. It's vital that we share with them, openly and sincerely. The Run required nothing from them except the willingness to observe, without any expectations in return. Their gift to us was already eminent – we needed to show them that our gift to them was too.

> Day 17 and 18
> Route: Anamosa, through Olin, to Mechanicsville, Iowa
> Weather: Very cold again. No rain.
> Comment: Newspapers, radio and television stations want our story. We're making progress. The strain on my body is terrible.

DAYS 17 & 18: SATURDAY & SUNDAY, MAY 18-19

Running through farmland continued to be the theme as I ran south toward Mount Vernon and Solon, Iowa. I ached more and more each day; my body felt the strain more than usual. When I sat down Sunday night to gather my thoughts, they were brief for I was soon fast asleep.

Day 19 and 20
Route: Mechanicsville to West Branch, Iowa.
Weather: Rain, with lightening
  Comment: Just traffic and more traffic.

DAYS 19 & 20: MONDAY & TUESDAY, MAY 20-21

As I ran toward Solon I met an interesting fellow. I called him the Lazarus Man because he raised himself back to life with the help of the Run. As I headed down a long stretch of country road, I saw in the distance someone walking to his mailbox. He was an older man, in his seventies, wearing bib overalls. As I came closer I saw him open the box and glance inside, then he looked up and spotted me jogging his way. He put the mail back in the box and waited. As I approached, he asked if I was "that fella running to Atlanta." When I said I was, he walked over and gave me the biggest bear hug I had ever received.

He backed away, obviously embarrassed. He told me he had never hugged a man before, and I said it was all right; we all need hugs. He went on to explain that his wife had died two years earlier and he had hidden inside his house ever since. He just hadn't cared about life anymore after his loss. When he read my story in the newspaper, however, he wanted to make sure he met me. He told me he had decided to live again, and that he wanted to thank me for helping to find his heart.

Stories like this added to the energy I remembered from the Twin Cities send-off. These stories kept me going stride after stride, step after step, day after day.

I went to bed Tuesday looking forward to the next day.

"When I worked for WCCO radio (in Minneapolis), I followed Terry all the way to Atlanta, two thousand miles, and talked with him on the radio one or two times each week. When I first met Terry, I had just completed running the Boston Marathon and I was really hurting. I thought Terry was crazy when he explained his plans to run a marathon each day – all the way to Atlanta. Yet, Terry made it to Atlanta, and he made a difference in the lives of those kids and families that he met and talked with along the way."

—John Williams

Host of Chicago's WGN Radio 720 midday show

CHAPTER 11

DAYS 21 THROUGH 30

Day 21
Route: West Branch to Iowa City, Iowa.
Weather: Some sunshine, a little wind
Comment: We had a home-cooked meal and slept in real beds. The media spent much of
the day with us.

DAY 21: WEDNESDAY, MAY 22

The start of the fourth week proved to be another wonderful day. I ran a total of twenty-seven miles, ending in Iowa City. After interviews with the *Iowa City Press Citizen*, KRNA-FM, WIRL-FM, and KGAN-TV, the team stayed overnight at the home of Linda and Jim, two new friends of the Run. Linda was a photographer with the *Iowa City Chronicle* newspaper, and a gracious host who made us feel comfortably at home. Jim, who worked in the real estate industry, told us how once for Mother's Day he walked one hundred miles in six days to give his mom a Mother's Day gift. Jim cooked dinner for us and Linda took us on a tour of the area. Both were wonderful hosts and the team appreciated the quality time, the taste of real food, and a night in real beds.

Day 22
Route: Iowa City to Ainsworth, Iowa.
Weather: Sun peaks from behind the clouds, but still cold and damp
Comment: The media follows us. Our equipment is falling apart; if things aren't being
stolen then they are breaking.

DAY 22: THURSDAY, MAY 23

On Thursday I ran thirty-five miles to Ainsworth in Southeastern Iowa. Upon arrival we entered a restaurant at a truck stop and were surprised to see a highlighted menu item: Terry's Run for Children and Single Parents.

Normally, we provided information on our Run the day we arrived, or media people received press kits from J. Marie a few days or a week prior to our appearance. Most media outlets had our daily Run schedule. Even so, it was a huge surprise to see myself on the dinner menu. I considered this another sign that we were having an impact, but I wondered, did it mean people were gravitating to our cause or were they just celebrating a physical feat?

As we gathered for the evening, Kim discussed with Chris how best to spend the few dollars we had left. J. Marie and the crew in the Twin Cities were still holding fundraisers, and the funds were sent to us for gas, food, and laundry. Still, we weren't rolling in money, and I was really feeling the pressure to raise money and set up more interviews.

Other logistical aspects of the Run were far from rosy. Mike's view of the trailer had become very negative. He mentioned numerous times that it was worthless from the beginning. The heater still didn't work, the water tank was broken, and we'd somehow lost a window. I woke up each morning with the weight of these problems on me and the knowledge that I needed to find a place for the crew to camp the coming evening. Add to that the PR work and the constant chore of calming the crew, and my day still wasn't done – I had to run at least twenty-seven miles.

I found it increasingly difficult to get motivated for a talk with the team members. I felt sorry for them. I am sure they were all doing their best, but they were frustrated. I could sympathize; I was frustrated too. However, in line with the old adage, I saw the glass as half-full while the kids saw it as half-empty.

I was reminded of Abraham Lincoln's anguish over his generals. Each general he appointed blamed a lack of resources for his failure to win battles. Lincoln kept changing generals, until finally appointing Ulysses S. Grant. Grant delighted Lincoln by deciding they could win with what they had. He was a problem solver. For instance, when Grant was given command of the Federal army, great numbers of Union cavalry were waiting in Washington for horses. Grant pointed out that those troops were taking up space and using up supplies. Either send the troops to him as foot soldiers, he suggested, or send them home and ship their supplies to the front lines. Lincoln was overjoyed with the practical choices. He sent the troops to Grant, despite the requests for manpower by other generals.

Those who say they can't accomplish anything without this or that simply don't make it. But those who focus on what they have, and how they can productively use what they have, succeed. I pondered how to pass this wisdom to kids raised in a consumer culture who believed that without certain possessions and environments their lives couldn't be made to work. I certainly didn't have the magic answer, but I did hope that by accomplishing the Run I would demonstrate how to succeed with what was available instead of not succeeding because of what wasn't.

This wasn't new wisdom. Plato, through Socrates, made the same observation more than two thousand years ago. In my opinion, children then had fewer options. Roman law allowed fathers to kill their sons if they didn't obey. Girls weren't allowed to participate in life arenas outside the home. And truthfully, things didn't improve dramatically over two millennia. Our wives and daughters had won the right to vote only in 1920, and brought the fight for economic and educational equality to a head in the late 60's and early 70's.

As I ran I wondered, who now was going to head up the fight for the fate of children. Do their struggles stem from a lack of interest in really doing something to help? Was their plight so pervasive and commonplace that we simply failed to notice? For kids' sake, we needed to solve this riddle. I wanted the Run to help foster a dialogue and lead to a solution.

Day 23
Route: Ainsworth to Mount Pleasant, Iowa.
Weather: Rain, yet again
   Comment: Lots of pain, and heavy traffic with impatient drivers.

DAY 23: FRIDAY, MAY 24

I planned to run more than seventy miles this coming weekend, passing through Mount Pleasant and eventually arriving in Burlington, Iowa. I recognized once again that my path to Atlanta was going to zigzag and that I would, at times, almost go through a part of a section of a state that I was near earlier. It was frustrating but at the same time the only way I could travel. I couldn't go on major expressways, so whatever road was available I was going to take; I had no choice. My pain was intense, but I had already come far. I didn't have far to go, I told myself. I would persist. I would push on. My body screamed, "Stop!" but my mind said, "Run on." I was reminded of the Bible verse *Matthew 26:41 (King James Version), which reads*, "The spirit is willing but the flesh is weak." I had to force my flesh to keep up with my spirit.

I overheard Chris tell a group of people that his dad was determined to finish this thing. He said it hurt him to see how I was hurting, but he realized there was no way I was going to stop running. Then, Chris spoke in a manner that not only made me feel proud, but told me how much he understood. He explained that there were twenty-three million kids and twelve million parents in single-parent homes, and that he could state from experience how tough it was for one parent to have to do it all. There were things missing in life for both the children and the parent. Kids, he said, may not be able to play sports after school because they didn't have someone to pick them up late, or the parent may forget to help with homework because he or she was too tired. A single parent, Chris admitted, misses out on many aspect of a normal adult social life. He said, "There is a need, and I think my dad is trying to make the voices of those thirty-five million heard."

He told the crowd that he hoped and prayed I wasn't pushing myself too hard, then, in characteristic teen-speak understatement, he added, "I mean, he's not a spring chicken."

Day 24
Route: Mount Pleasant, through New London, to Burlington, Iowa
Weather: Cloudy and mild
Comment: Warm beds and dry clothes for everyone. The team is tired and cold.

DAY 24: SATURDAY, MAY 25

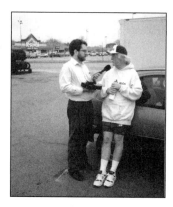

I will never forget what happened in Burlington, Iowa. We were interviewed by *The Hawkeye* and three radio stations. The radio station manager, Chip Giannettino, opened up his home to the team. Chip often took his family camping and he did so that night to make room for us. He knew we were wet and cold and probably running out of gas, both figuratively and literally. It was a welcome break for everyone. The past three weeks were suffused with cold and rain, and the constant pounding on my body was wearing me down. As I finished the day's run, the thought of a nice, warm shower was mixed with a delightful realization: Chip's favor would enable me to keep my annual ritual of watching the Indianapolis 500 race.

It also gave the team members an opportunity to rest and be quiet. Charlie was quiet as well and obviously not feeling his best. We all had been closely watching Charlie and trying to make sure he didn't become exhausted running with me on the highways. So it was becoming obvious that the stress of not sleeping in his own bed and being in familiar surroundings was contributing to his lethargy. I reminded myself and the others to keep a close eye on him. Kim's spirits improved when her mother arrived for a visit.

Overall, it was quite a relief to see everyone unwind and find a bit of quiet solitude for his or her beaten-up spirits.

Unfortunately, the brief respite of Chip's gift had a downside. I had hoped it would bring a new light to the eyes of the crew. Instead, it seemed to serve as a stark contrast to the hardships of the trailer and reminded the team members how pleasant it would be back home on their own beds, in their own lives, and with their own friends. Even though we were focused on helping thirty-five million people, we all were beginning to realize that the actual passion and emotion for this trek really only resided in me. I found myself hoping again that the team members would stick it out. However, in my heart I felt loneliness, a premonition that soon I would be without them. I prayed it wouldn't be so, but sometimes a well-deserved break only makes things harder for those not fully committed.

I reminded myself that I was probably being too hard on these youngsters. My commitment was earned through years and years of growing pains and hard-fought maturity. The kids hadn't had those experiences yet. They were still learning and growing, and I needed to continue learning and growing as well. No matter what happened, I felt blessed for the support, love, and dedication the team had given.

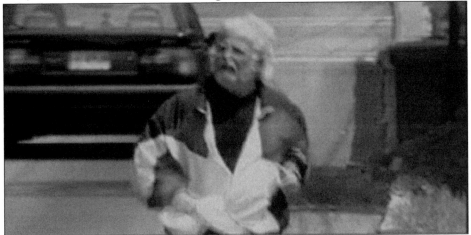

Day 25
Route: Burlington to Media, Ill.
Weather: Cold as usual.
Comment: Traffic continues to be a problem. I'm careful not to become someone's target. The dampness permeates every part of me.

DAY 25: SUNDAY, MAY 26

I arrived in Rosedale, Illinois, after a remarkable forty-eight miles. I questioned then (and still question now) how this was possible. The pain was subsiding somewhat, though, and each day I started to feel stronger. That week I planned to run as much as possible, hoping for warmer weather. Kicking it off with nearly fifty miles in a single day inspired me. If I could cover that distance in one day, anything seemed possible.

A less positive realization was that runners can also become a target of opportunity for cars. I had to jump into ditches alongside the road many times as cars and trucks came by. Some people apparently just couldn't stand to share the road with anyone who wasn't traveling by vehicle. Those close calls both terrified and angered me. They challenged my resolve to continue, but at the same time strengthened my determination to continue and not be run off the road by anyone.

I usually ran on the shoulder, against traffic, so I could see what's coming. Sometimes, however, that side wasn't good for running or had no shoulder at all, and I had to run with my back to the traffic. Once, in Iowa, a car actually left the road to chase me down on the shoulder. It came within a fraction of an inch of hitting me – the only reason he missed was my quick dive into a ditch. Another day, when I was running against the traffic, a driver deliberately moved onto the shoulder and drove straight at me. Again, I tumbled and escaped the pick-up's wheels. The driver's intent was obvious, but the police were helpless. They simply told me that some people don't like joggers.

Maybe these people just wanted to get my attention. If so, mission accomplished. Maybe they were angry with others and I was just an easy target for their aggression. Or perhaps they thought their actions were funny. Regardless of why they did it, I wondered how many other people they made miserable with their senseless acts, mean actions, and depraved sense of humor. Life is fragile enough without being subjected to threats from perfect strangers. These people had the gift of life but didn't appreciate it enough to respect it in others. Was it any wonder our families and schools were under assault? I had always strived to understand human nature, but I couldn't make any sense out of deliberately trying to hit someone with a vehicle. I guess I was fair game to those kinds of people and if that says something about humanity it's a sad commentary. At times I think our culture has turned upon itself. We cater to the childish inclinations of adults rather than the adult preparation of children. There are malicious people in every community, whether rural or urban. Just as one rotten apple can spoil the whole barrel, so too can one or two rotten human beings sour the reputation of a whole community.

Anyway, as of May 26 I had managed to dodge every vehicle. So far, so good.

In contrast to the drivers who tried to run me off the road, some people gave me a wide berth, either trying to be nice or trying to just ignore me. In conversations about kids of single parents I was sometimes given the same wide berth. Some people are embarrassed by the topic or they want to change the subject to something they think they can deal with. Others refuse to hear anything that might shake their defense mechanisms or challenge their beliefs. At some level they must be aware that even mere acknowledgement can have profound, life-altering effects. In many conversations about single parents, it was insinuated to me that single parents are in situations of their own making. It's their fault. Maybe this is true at times, but not usually. Stereotypes like this help no one, and regardless of the cause or fault behind single parenthood, the kids are still left to suffer for the actions of adults.

Fault is a relative term of judgment that does the kids no good if, by deeming the parent blameworthy, the community deprives the children of its support and resources. The latter is short sighted indeed, as these kids are part of the community's future.

Sadly, there are too many people who want to run this topic off the road.

Nevertheless, during the Run the stories in the newspapers were heartwarming. So were those moments when someone told me that now they understood, they considered my message and planned to do what they could for the children of single-parent families. Each time I heard this response I knew I was further ahead than when I had started. I felt like Johnny Appleseed, sowing those ideas one person at a time. Of course, I never knew whether the coming ground was fertile or fallow – I just knew I had to spread the seeds as broadly as I could.

Day 26
Route: Media to Roseville, Illinois.
Weather: Cold and rainy
  Comment: The look on team members' faces tells the story: this is not fun any more.

DAY 26: MONDAY, MAY 27

Monday was another long, rainy, cold day. I looked up at the sky every few steps and asked silently, where was the sun we were promised? My back began giving me problems and despite the high of the previous day's accomplishment, I felt lonely and emotionally down. I attributed the minor depression to the weather, as if the sun could save me but had chosen to forsake me. I needed to remember that the answer resided inside me, not outside. The trailer was still providing very little warmth or power, though, and that contributed to the difficulty of feeling good each day. The rest of the team was really starting to look depressed. Again, I wondered how long it would be before other team members decided to go home. They didn't talk to me about it, but I could see it in their eyes. I tried pep talks, talking about the cause, the purpose, insisting that we could do it, that we needed to look at the positive side. I also pointed out that this is a challenge they could meet that would make them proud and give them wonderful stories to tell. Still, their enthusiasm was definitely on the wane.

Nonetheless, despite the cold weather and ceaseless problems with the trailer, Monday did bring a good experience. As I was running down a narrow road between farms, a farmer and his son stood waiting at the end of their driveway. I had become accustomed to this; it seemed like half the world had waited for me at the ends of various driveways. This particular family had seen my story and picture in their local newspaper, and when they saw my route took me past their place, they decided to come out to see me. The son, James, asked if I was Terry, the runner. He was handicapped and had to support himself on a walker as he stood next to his dad. He said he wanted to help other kids, and gave me two dollars from his savings. His mom had died five years earlier and James and his dad lived alone. James wanted to meet me and give me a hug – so we hugged, and I thanked his dad for the opportunity to meet two new friends. They really made my day. But I was happier that my Run and our meeting had helped make their day.

Day 27
Route: Roseville, through London Mills, to Farmington, Ill.
Weather: Very damp
Comment: Our friend Michael Durant reminds us that we are accomplishing an
  impossible task. The team is exhausted from the cold and wet.

DAY 27: SUNDAY, MAY 28

One of the greatest pleasures of running on the road was the sound of birds chirping, as if to say, "Keep on running, Terry, keep on running." They provided the rhythmic beat of their own singing metronomes and kept me in the running groove.

In Peoria, I ran past the *Spirit of Peoria* stern-wheeler paddleboat. The sound of the paddle wheel going round and round provided its own rhythm. So many beats, so different, all encouraged me to keep running and keep the steps following one after another. I saw people riding in boats. They were sitting down, missing out on this natural rhythm of Mother Nature. As my body moved in tune with the Earth, they merely glided effortlessly to the hum of outboard motors. I wished I could convey to them the joys of running.

The *Peoria Daily Journal*, WMVD-TV, and WEEK-TV were on hand when the team arrived. I had an interview with radio station WMBD, then was interviewed by various groups at the Oasis Center. I was particularly moved by these good people. Michael Durant joined us – he was filming a documentary of my Run for the Children Are Forever Foundation and MegaMarathon '96. I was asked how the Run was going, how I felt, and the ever-present question: what did I hope to accomplish? I talked about 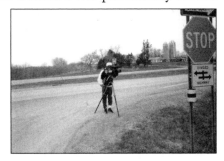 the goal of raising awareness of the plight of kids in single-parent families. I talked about the Run, both its joys and its loneliness. I recounted, once again, the Terry Fox story. I talked about my hopes for good things to happen for the foundation as a result of the Run, my hope that the foundation could do good things for kids and parents.

I talked about how, when my wife died, I was left with three small children and no housekeeping skills. In retrospect, it was kind of embarrassing to admit that I had to learn to cook. I related my double whammy of losing my job just a couple of days after my wife died. I explained through my favorite baseball metaphor how I had stepped up to the plate of life with two strikes against me. I talked about how tough a time I had had, and that strike three had come in the form of deep depression.

I told the interviewers about Terry Fox, and how inspiring his run had been to me. He had just graduated from high school when cancer was discovered on his right knee. With the loss of his leg, he decided to try to help by raising people's awareness. He decided to run across Canada. And after he got started, this one young man had everyone in Canada waking up with one question on their minds, "Where is Terry Fox today?"

I was one of those people, in my home in the U.S., watching this saga unfold. I watched as his mission grew bigger and bigger. Though cancer cut short Terry Fox's effort, he had literally given his life for others. He had set out to raise one million dollars, and his valiant effort touched people throughout Canada, the U.S., and beyond. By the end of his Run, Terry raised over $24 million! And now, his legacy has grown to over $400 million.

Terry Fox had an emotional and inspirational impact on many people. One of those people was me. Terry Fox's inner strength struck an important chord in me, and I hoped I could push with as much effort as he had. In Peoria, I explained to my interviewers that, like Terry, I wasn't a runner. I was a man who Ran to help children.

People were also interested in the logistics of the Run. I shared Chris's job with them, how he tracked my distance each day and monitored what I ate and drank. I was burning over 6,000 calories a day, and Chris was feeding me every forty minutes, as well as bringing me water and a special sports liquid every twenty minutes. He forced more and more bananas into me as my body craved potassium when I pushed it to extremes. Somehow, in the midst of this constant attention to my health, Chris also did a tremendous amount of driving back and forth. He often acted as the advance scout, going on ahead to talk with the media or whoever else might want to talk with us in the next town.

The interviewers also asked what life was like after I became a single parent. I think they were searching for more affirmation that our mission was truly significant. I explained how adult friends had drifted away as they sensed that I had somehow become different. Having no spouse often means not being invited to gatherings anymore. I became lonely and depressed. At night I had no one to turn to. Many people can't understand the importance of having someone to simply say, "You're doing okay," until that person is no longer around. When my wife died and I became the kids' sole caregiver, I became different. Where I should have been half of a whole, I was just one half. It was a very lonely existence, and sometimes the problems just seemed too hard to deal with.

This provided an opportunity to describe the metaphor of the single-parent marathon. When my wife died, I had three kids in three different schools. All at once I was the person who had to attend to things such as sick calls from the nurse at school and making sure the kids got to evening piano lessons. I didn't always know what to do. I might forget to say goodnight or forget that I needed to make supper, or even forget to say, "I love you." And in addition to the direct support, I had to cover the indirect. I still had to make the money to pay the mortgage and put food on the table. I absolutely could not afford to be sick.

I went on to explain my sense that we will have a lost generation coming of age unless we can help parents and their kids, and keep the kids from prematurely becoming parents themselves, let alone single parents. I asked the question why, in this country, we say our kids are the future, yet we don't have laws to reflect that philosophy. I asked again why we don't have a Secretary of Children. Kids must be enabled to believe they can succeed. If there's something they want to do with their lives, they just need to set about doing it, set their goals, and act on them. They don't need any special reasons – they just need to believe.

I told the interviewers that during the trek some people had called me crazy, or referred to me as "Forrest Gump." Some said I was a Nike commercial – "Just do it!" I laughed and told them that although I trained in Nikes, I was running in New Balances. Bill Rudkin in Connecticut, who had heard about the Run from his friend, Rick Marklund, made my shirts, shorts, and outerwear. His company specialized in running clothes—even custom underwear to make running easier on men and boys. Bill had clothes designed especially for the Run and paid for his gifts out of his own pocket.

I learned that Bill even went to the president of New Balance and had shoes made for the team. The shoes were the New Balance "999." Each team member had a pair to go along with his or her specially-made and designed clothing. I received ten pairs and changed my shoes two to four times each day, depending on the weather and the road conditions. Not once did I have foot problems; no blisters whatsoever. The New Balance 999s had extremely fine support and more room inside than most running shoes. I imagined that few shoes, if any, could take the abuse I gave my footwear. They withstood terrific pounding on uneven surfaces all day, and went through torrential downpours before moving straight into oven-baked one hundred degree temperatures, all in a matter of hours. Bill Rudkin and New Balance were life savers. Bill is an extraordinary friend.

I also took the opportunity to mention Wigwam Socks. Like New Balance, Wigwam supported us with donated clothing, and their socks were an important factor in the survival of my feet. It was extraordinary to see absolutely no blisters, given the constant stress of the roadside terrain I ran on each day.

Another sponsor was Dominos Pizza even though they knew pizza could not be part of my nutrition regimen. They sponsored a *Children Are Forever Day* in Minnesota and generously donated a percentage of their receipts to the Run.

The Peoria interviewers also asked Chris for his thoughts. He told them the toughest thing about his mom dying was that it happened a week before his eighth birthday. Also, like me, he had become involuntarily different. His friends excluded him and didn't want to play with him anymore. He shared other details with the media, describing what it was like to grow up with only one parent. Then, he told them that he had dropped out of college for two quarters so he could help me with this Run because he believed in the cause. He mentioned how difficult it had been for him on the Run so far, being away from friends and having to put the needs of the Run above everything else in his life. He likened the trip to an emotional roller coaster, with the rises and falls each day often beginning with arguments. Chris said he could be in a great mood one day, and not know what to do with the next mood swing.

He also said the Run was really helping him personally. He had felt out of focus before, barely making it through high school. In the past he had been afraid to talk with people on the phone whereas now, forced to do so on the Run, he had become more confident and capable. To him, the Run experience was like an awakening. Overall he saw it as an adventure, and he felt he had learned a great deal. He was proud to explain to the media how much self-confidence he had developed, and how much he felt he had already grown as a result of this trip.

Of course, it went without saying that I was proud of the job Chris was doing, and particularly of his growth as a young man. For the first time I could remember, he was able to assert himself and, thus, insert himself into a wide range of discussions, including the interactions with the media, the team, and the tremendous variety of people we met on the Run.

Michael also interviewed the crewmembers. Kim started out by telling him she really believed in the Run. She talked about how she became involved – she had wanted to learn about public relations and thought this would be a perfect training event. Also, she wanted to be in at the ground level before Children Are Forever went big. Kim also stated something I had not been willing to admit, though it seemed prophetic. She said that, though we had been met in many cities with a great deal of interest, it may have been more for the runner than the cause. She didn't see any interest developing at a wider, national level, certainly not the outpouring Terry Fox received during his Run – not even a trickle in comparison. Despite her early motivation, she didn't really see Children Are Forever making it big. The trip had been hard for her physically, and she could tell she was getting tired because of the negative ways she was beginning to react to Chris and me.

Chris's comments confirmed Kim's feelings. He admitted he suspected that Kim and Mike were thinking it was time to leave. Kim didn't seem happy to him; he said she had lost the joy she had first brought to the Run. One minute she smiled and joked, the next she might bite his head off; the constant conflict was driving him crazy. Likewise, Mike hadn't gotten to the point of being actively upset, but he wasn't enthusiastic any more. Chris also said he was afraid the others' attitude had begun to affect me and could jeopardize the Run. He hadn't shared this with me before because he hadn't wanted to add to my burden.

Because I spent so much time on the road, I was only vaguely aware of the dissent. I had been too tired and inwardly withdrawn to fully recognize and deal with it. I realized that if I were ever to do this again, I would still need young people, but that I would also need a mature adult to manage the younger crewmembers. I needed someone who could motivate them, cheer them, and also make decisions based on the good of the Run, while still taking into consideration their individual personalities. As the runner, I just couldn't handle these critical tasks.

Though the interviews in Peoria with Michael were somewhat negative, they probably brought some relief to the crew. One third of the way through, the Run had become far more difficult than any of us had imagined. The cold rain and strong winds had taken their toll. Everyone was tired and cold. The trailer still didn't work well, and the hot water still wasn't hot. Just finding a place to park the trailer each night was a major undertaking, and people had stolen things out of the cars and truck. My wallet and checkbook were gone. The brakes on the cars were going bad. It seemed as though a version of Murphy's Law was at work, and the metaphor for single parenthood was becoming excruciatingly real. And I planned on running almost thirty miles the next day.

Just when it seemed nothing could go right, we were given an amazing surprise – the Holiday Inn provided us with free rooms in Peoria and at our next destination. I guess God felt it was about time we came in from the rain and enjoyed hot baths and warm beds.

Day 28
Route: Farmington, through Hanna City and Belle View, to Peoria, Ill.
Weather: A quick glimpse of the sun, but still cold and damp.
Comment: An upbeat day. People are supportive, making the pain bearable.

DAY 28: WEDNESDAY, MAY 29

Some mornings were just made for Psalms. One of my favorites is Psalms 118:24, which reads *Today is the day the Lord hath made; let us rejoice and be glad in it.* That was how I felt that Wednesday, mainly because there was no rain. We left Peoria, Illinois, and headed for Springfield under full sunlight. Even if it's just for a little while, dry weather made everything feel better. Nonetheless, I felt tired. I ran twenty-nine miles, and each one seemed longer than the usual mile. The highway I traveled had very little shoulder, and I constantly had to jump aside for oncoming traffic. Fortunately, Charlie rode in the trailer, as he had been most of the time the past few days. He still wasn't feeling well and just wanted to sleep. I think he was homesick and longed for his favorite chair at home in Minneapolis. I couldn't blame him.

Despite the scary drivers, for the first time it seemed that most people on the road were excited and truly aware of MegaMarathon '96. Car and truck horns honked and people waved as they drove by. The gestures really felt good. It showed the hearts of people as they learned about our cause; and for others, it simply meant they were interested in this feat of feet and wanted to show their support. It showed me it is worthwhile to attempt the difficult, to challenge one's self to achieve what is perceived as impossible without being disheartened.

I also met another person who really lifted my spirits. While running, I came across a fellow sitting in a chair just off the highway. He was an artist of a special order – he painted landscapes on the sides of barns. For his current piece he was painting what he saw in the area around the barn. We talked for a long time about the community and his life experiences. As I readied myself to resume the Run, he said he had planned on painting the Coca-Cola logo, a very typical adornment for barn artistry. However, he changed his mind during our conversation, and was going to paint the *"Children Are Forever"* logo instead.

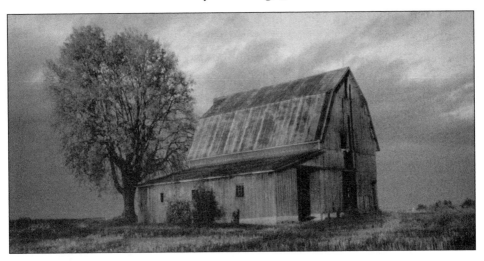

Day 29
Route: Peoria to Pekin, on our way to Springfield, Ill.
Weather: Cold but no rain.
   Comment: Exhausted and disenchanted, the team leaves. Only Chris and I remain.

DAY 29: THURSDAY, MAY 30

Some distance running beyond Peoria, Chris and Michael drove up along side me. The sky was overcast, a gloomy portrait of what was to come. Chris and Michael insisted I stop and pulled me aside, sitting me down in the car. I knew something was wrong, but my focus was really on running and dealing with the next segment of the road. Chris dropped the news bluntly, sensing that straightforward was the best choice: Mike and Kim had decided to return to Minnesota.

I was saddened but not really surprised.

The question was now, who would drive the trailer? We considered several options. Maybe Andy or Jason could come back down, or someone else. Maybe I could drive the trailer ahead and have Chris take me back to the day's starting point; then I could run to the trailer with a little more knowledge of the intervening road. I think it was Michael who came up with

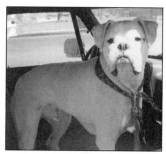

the best solution: send the trailer back with Kim and Mike, pack down the car, and try to find a hotel that would comp us a room every night. That seemed to make as much, if not more sense, than any other option.

We also decided Kim and Mike would take Charlie back as well, since he wouldn't do well in a cramped space in the packed car, especially with the hot weather forecast ahead of us. He could stay with friends until the end of the Run.

So, we packed the car with everything we could make fit and the remainder went back in the trailer. Kim and Mike drove off for the Twin Cities and Chris sat with me by the side of the road. It was transition time. We knew we had to get it together physically, spiritually, logistically, and rationally. As we pondered the immediate future, we experienced a strange phenomenon of timing. The kids who were leaving hadn't yet learned the power of a positive mental attitude. They still allowed the negative to dominate when they were challenged. As they drove off, the sun broke through the clouds, as if it were finally allowed to shine where it would be appreciated.

Day 30
Route: Pekin toward Greenview, Ill.
Weather: Sunny and warm (finally!)
Comment: My body is in major pain. Chris and I are exhausted.

DAY 30: FRIDAY, MAY 31

We headed toward Springfield, Illinois, the state capital. We also realized that by the Run's end, Chris would put thirteen thousand miles on the car to my two thousand miles on foot. Chris had called the Governor's office and asked for an opportunity to meet him June 2, but by the end of May, we hadn't received a response.

For the first time, we had to find a hotel willing to donate a room or we knew our accommodations would be the front seats of the car. Chris tried a number of hotels in the Springfield area and finally was given a complimentary room at the Sky Harbour Lodge. What a blessing!

My ankles were really beginning to hurt and I wondered if perhaps I had damaged them more severely than expected. I knew I was subjecting them to a staggering amount of constant wear and tear, but I started to think I might have caused a more specific, chronic injury. For a few mornings now I had had trouble putting on my socks because of pain in my heels. Then again, I told myself, I shouldn't be surprised by anything at this point.

"Terry Hitchcock's story – from the death of his young wife to his mega-marathon run to his endeavors in business and charity – epitomizes what life at its most fundamental level is all about: overcoming obstacles ... and helping others do the same. Only Terry discovered what many sadly miss – that God has a sovereign plan for each one of us, that He provides the supernatural power to overcome, and that it's all for His glory and our good."

—David Wheaton

A professional tennis player, radio talk show host, and author of *University of Destruction*.

CHAPTER 12

REFLECTIONS

When ships sailed the oceans three hundred to five hundred years ago, they referred to the "Middle Passage," the time between the beginning and the end of a voyage when there was nothing in sight but the vast expanse of the sea. No land. No islands. Just water. The next land they encountered would either be the land of their destination, the land they had left (because they turned back), or the bottom of the ocean floor, because they sank. Chris and I were now in a similar position. Fortunately, we were on land, not water. The only thing that could make us turn back would be losing our resolve. The thing that could sink us would be a car or truck running me over, but I had dodged them so far and I was confident I could continue to do so. We were determined not to lose our resolve. We knew our destination. We knew we had to continue. We decided to deal with any hurdles and not to worry about them in advance.

It began to dawn on Chris and me that we might have to sleep in the car some nights if the hotels didn't work out. The fundraisers were barely keeping up with our food, gas and routine expenses, and we simply had not budgeted for hotels. We had planned to camp in the trailer. We decided to give sleeping in the car a try. Sleep in the car required sitting up because the back seat and trunk were fully loaded with supplies and goods necessary for the trip. I felt we could do some sleeping sitting up if we absolutely had to. I was more worried about the humid and hot weather as we headed farther south.

We were confused and depressed. The Run that had started with such promise and celebration and enthusiastic support had now left Chris and I confused and depressed. The rundown Oldsmobile Chris drove had more than two hundred thousand miles on it and we still had more than one thousand miles to go to reach Atlanta. This moment in our trek was difficult to wrestle with. Chris and I now were alone on the highway with no support vehicle, no trailer, and no team — just the two of us against some rather difficult elements. We wondered how we would get through each day.

Chris now had to wear six hats. He would have to feed me, take care of the car, do the laundry, keep the daily records of the Run collecting daily

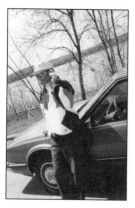

mileage and road conditions, and work closely with the media, calling television and radio stations, talking with the local and national newspapers, setting up meetings and scheduling interviews. In addition to all of this, he now had to do everything else that came under the catchall of miscellaneous. He had to make certain that I was surviving each mile, each day, eating every forty minutes, drinking every twenty minutes. Chris wondered if he could do it; I prayed that he could.

Saying goodbye is not easy in most situations. It certainly wasn't easy to see my team go home. They too were sad but knew that they had to leave. It had not been easy for any of us. The weather was cold and wet and our equipment and supplies were not adequate. As Chris and I watched the rest of the team turn toward home and drive away, I wondered what more I could have done to make it less difficult for everyone, to overcome the dampness and the daily struggles that became too much for them. What could I have done to prevent the scene that, to any outside observer, must have looked like two pathetic guys in an old car abandoned by the side of the road.

There is no greater joy than beating adversity, but maybe this just wasn't the right time or the right fight for these kids. But, I at least had a hope that they had taken something away from their month on this trip to give them new tools and new resolve to beat whatever adversity may throw at them down the road of life.

Chris and I could not turn away from our face-to-face with adversity. We knew it would be a struggle for me to continue putting one foot in front of the other. But we had one piece of strength not often given to people in adversity. We had a calendar date – July 15, seven weeks away – by which we knew it would be over. It wasn't as if we had to do this for months or years. People who run life's daily marathons without an end in sight are the real heroes. We chose this freely. We asked ourselves what is another seven weeks given the rigors of the past eighteen months? We looked at each other and laughed.

I called my friend Peter Jessen on the phone. He is another single parent, a man raising three young boys. I told him we were sitting by the side of the road laughing. He laughed with us, saying his graduate school professor, Peter Berger, wrote in his book *Redeeming Laughter* that nothing should be taken so seriously that it supersedes the capacity for laughter. Laughter can be redemptive. "You have laughed," Jessen said. "You have suspended the serious world. You have passed that test."

Peter assured us, though, the seriousness would return. Those with woes need to laugh, whether with belly laughs or giggles or anything in between, if they are to survive what can be a mean and unfriendly world. All the great clowns of our century, Charlie Chaplin, Buster Keaton, Victor Borge, Laurel and Hardy, Abbott and Costello, Martin and Lewis, Hope and Crosby, Burns and Allen, Bill Cosby, and many more, have played characters that faced troubles and persecution and hard times. How did they survive? With laughter.

"So," Peter told me, "look at your pro-motional poster. It's a picture of you and your kids, your dog, and some balloons. Clowns. ... You started with that marvelous sensibility. Don't stop. Keep being clowns. Only they can survive when life really gets serious, for they can see the humor, the spark of life, in even the darkest corner. So," he said, "pick yourselves

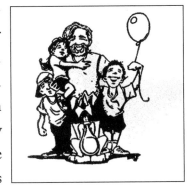

up again, laugh, and go on as you always have, and as you will always do, because that is you. The tragic character falls and lies there, stoically accepting reality, and death. The clown laughs, says there is another reality – life – and gets up and goes on."

Peter laughed again, saying he was picturing us sitting on the side of the road, by an old, crammed-to-the-roof car, with a thousand miles to go. He asked how he could possibly feel sorry for us when we would have such good material for jokes and campfire stories in the years after the Run was done. "You laughed before," he reminded me, "and you will laugh tomorrow."

I had to smile as I pictured him sitting in his comfortable chair, neither cold and damp nor sweaty and tired. In my mind's eye, I envisioned him preaching to me at the South Pole, naked. He looked funny. He sounded funny. And I knew he was right. Humor is what I often used to help my kids through the darkest of times as well as to help clients who had hired me to help them solve problems. They couldn't see straight until they had a smile on their face. I had to get them to smile. Now it was my turn to find humor in adversity. This is exactly the driving force behind the profoundly wise 1999 Academy Award-winning film, *Life is Beautiful*, in which a father finds laughter and humor in a World War II concentration camp and uses it to save his son's life.

I looked at my son Chris and I was thankful for this other source of strength. He was with his dad. He knew what it meant to me. I am certain he wanted to get back to his friends. But loving me as only a son can, he stayed. Chris put up with things others would not, not because I am Terry Hitchcock, but because I am his dad; I am family. The same is true for Jason and Teri Sue. I imagined it must have been that way during the settlement of the West. It must have been a time when kids and their families did things to make it work, not because they wanted to, but because the kids and their parents were suffering the same hardships. They learned they could share hardships and build something. They sat around campfires, sang songs, laughed and told stories about what happened earlier that hadn't *seemed* funny. Chris was learning the same lesson, that it is not the hardship that counts but how one responds to it and what one builds out of the hardship. What greater gift could my son receive than what he was learning on this trip?

So, it was difficult moments like these that proved to me why it all matters, why it is meaningful to go on, what it means to be more than a father and a role model, and why the generations need each other and feed so positively off each other. Chris assured me that we would do just fine and that God would be present as He always had been, and that what was important was not what happened to us, but how we handled it. At that moment my heart swelled with pride to hear the lessons Sue and I had so carefully nurtured in our children now come back as inspiration and motivation to me at a time when I needed it.

So, as the rest of the team headed back to the Twin Cities, Chris and I sat in the front seat of our old car, staring at each other with blank faces that turned to grins. The back seat and trunk were stacked with supplies. We wondered again where we would sleep and how I was going to get the nourishment and support I needed to make it through each day. As we surveyed our plight, we couldn't help ourselves. Our grins broke into laughter. We roared. Instead of tears we found laughter, gales of redemptive laughter.

I had an epiphany that day. I realized why so many people beat great odds. They laugh with God, however they define Him, rather than get angry at Him. They use His strength for their efforts rather than waste their own strength cursing Him. I was reminded of a poet's comment that God "laughs over the waves." Certainly, we were a small, tiny, little ship of purpose floating on a sea of time in unknown, uncharted waters, a sea that stretched before us not in watery miles but in weeks. Seven weeks.

But, of course! I got out of the car. I started to run. Poor Chris. He had to ride in the stuffed car. I got to enjoy the sun, the warm wind, and the great outdoors. I laughed some more.

Back home, our team and other supporters were holding a variety of fund-raisers and wiring the proceeds to us so we could continue to meet our expenses. There was plenty of action going on behind the scenes. Chris and I continued on our way. I nursed my sore muscles, both of us carved out our plans and strategies for each day. The real heartbeat of the Run, dozens of involved volunteers and friends back in the Twin Cities, created a lifeline through which they pumped the support, enthusiasm and funds that enabled us to go on. These people were dedicated to seeing this MegaMarathon '96 through to its completion. But there wasn't enough money for motels, and even if there had been, I would have been hard pressed to spend it that way. We needed so much else that seemed vastly more important.

Part of the success of these efforts to raise money was attributable to over two dozen wonderful children who came together, through the urging of Otis Courtney and Marcus Knight, as the Children Are Forever choir, blending together their beautiful voices. Otis and Marcus gathered more than two-dozen children to form a choir to sing at fundraisers and to represent children everywhere. Their performance at fundraisers was special and their support was valuable to me every day on the road. We raised money by putting our hands in plaster of Paris and then selling our "hands" to moms and dads. We had gatherings where everyone brought their dogs and called the event a Bow Wow gathering. Everything we did was fun and the community always joined in. Many times we met at the Mall of America and people gathered around our events all day long. Just remembering the choir's voices and their love and their expressed appreciation for what I was trying to accomplish helped me during the tough times. Thanks, kids.

We also had supporters for a day, as I called them. In town after town, day after day, week after week, these people, who had been deeply touched by our mission, came forward to aid us.

Meanwhile J. Marie and her firm, Nemer, Fieger and Associates in Minneapolis, continued to work their public relations magic. They pulled the logistics of the news coverage together for the Run, coordinated the fundraisers, acted as cheerleaders for the workers in Minneapolis, kept us on our agenda, pulled rabbits out of their hats and proved the validity of their leading-edge thinking about how to market the Run. To all with whom they came in contact, whether in the Twin Cities or on the road, they brought positive news and lifted spirits.

In the midst of all of the chaos, Chris never lost sight of the fact that it was extremely important to feed me on a precise schedule. My life literally depended on it. I was scheduled to eat every forty minutes and to drink at least every twenty minutes. My food was special, as was what I drank. To run more than two thousand miles I couldn't just drink water. In fact, water wouldn't have gotten me there. My liquids were a mixture of various powdered ingredients mixed with water. I took heavy doses of vitamins, a horse-pill sized amino acid supplement, and a long list of other substances designed to meet my body's needs.

Each day I burned more than six thousand calories. Chris drove what we now called our pace car and monitored my needs and symptoms. He drove about two or three miles ahead to check out the condition of the highway, to make certain that there was room for me to run, and to see what towns and cities lay ahead. He made sure that he always drove back so I wouldn't miss either my fluid break or my food break. He also provided ice packs for my knees and other achy spots. He had to pack the car so that the many changes of clothes, towels, food, ice packs and medical supplies were available and ready each day.

Chris had already experienced the daily marathon of life as a child in a single-parent household. Now he had taken on the adult role through our extended metaphor. He was amazing.

"Music has and will always be an important part of my life. Music is the thread throughout all our lives. It is the basis of our being, of creating the magic. Terry's run and the support of Chris, Jason and Teri Sue is a story that all kids and their parents should be fully aware of. Their story is one of courage and one of passion for helping others. As in music, Terry's Run depicts the heart and soul of the rhythms in life and its beauty."

—Jordis Unga

A rock star that has performed in front of a multitude of thousands, touring originally with her band, "The Fighting Tongs" with lead guitarist Jason Hitchcock. The band performed in the concert tour "Riverfest," along with Twisted Sister, Anthrax, Sevendust and Damage Plan. She was a contestant on CBS's *Star Search* and a finalist on CBS's *Rock Star*

CHAPTER 13

DAYS 31 THROUGH 40

Day 31
Route: On the road to Springfield, arriving at Greenview, Ill.
Weather: Sunny
Comment: Holiday Inn stepped up. Thank you! Someone is always there when you need them most.

DAY 31: SATURDAY, JUNE 1

We'd met with wonderful hospitality along the way, ranging from individuals who welcomed us into their homes to inns and motels that provided free rooms for a night. But Holiday Inn did something that, after one of our lowest moments, restored our spirits and brought a new sense of possibility. They offered us complimentary rooms for the rest of the Run!

Once it became just Chris and me and the front seat of the Oldsmobile – no trailer, no tent, nothing in which to lie down – we had to get creative. We had stayed free at a Holiday Inn once before and Chris suggested we try it again. He drove us back along the route to a hotel he had noticed earlier. The manager there listened to my story and decided to make a difference. But he did more than just provide us with a room and breakfast at no cost. This fine innkeeper presented us with a letter of introduction we could use at other Holiday Inns as we continued.

To adequately describe his generosity, I have to mix my stories, metaphors, and parables. Holiday Inn shared with us the meaning of the story of the Good Samaritan. The company did not hang "No Room at the Inn" signs; instead, they gave us shelter and food, and asked nothing in return, not even publicity. Holiday Inn wasn't an original sponsor – when we started off with the trailer, we didn't think we would ever need a hotel, and they didn't know we existed. Yet the hotel chain became a real friend, a self-appointed sponsor. Even though the company's focus was on the Summer Olympics, they found the willingness to be Good Samaritans to us and to our cause. They befriended strangers, just as in the parable. They made room at their inn. What a miracle! Though they didn't ask for it, they certainly deserved special recognition.

Day 32
Route: Greenview to Springfield, Ill.
Weather: Sunny, again.
  Comment: We are inspired visiting in front of Lincoln's Tomb.

DAY 32: SUNDAY, JUNE 2

Today the sun continued to shine. Chris and I often thought of our team, the team members who returned home. We were getting accustomed to the fact that from now on it was just the two of us. The back seat and trunk of the Oldsmobile were stuffed with supplies. The precious letter from the Holiday Inn, and no concerns about where we would sleep each night, put grins on both our faces.

I needed to be able to grin, as did Chris. His responsibilities had increased far beyond the point of reasonable expectation. Whenever we assessed our situation we looked at each other and broke out laughing again. There was indeed a redemptive healing aspect of being able to look at the bright side, not seeing ourselves as victims, but rather seeing the new challenges, new mountains to climb, and raising our personal bar and making the effort to jump over it. I again realized the truth of how those who beat great odds do so: they laugh with God rather than get angry with Him. They tap into His power rather than fight it. They believe in being, they appreciate the gift of life, they allow the strength within to manifest itself externally, then they use it to pull through the hardship at hand. We would do the same.

When we got to Springfield, Illinois, WICS-TV and NBC TV were there to meet us. They spent a great deal of time talking about Children Are

Forever and the focus and passion of the Run. The NBC interviewer told me I had opened doors that had never been open before. I hoped he was right. He filmed Chris and me on the highway and on my visit to Lincoln's tomb, a visit I had long been looking forward to.

I was emotional, standing before the tomb. I believed I understood how Lincoln must have felt as he persevered through the ordeal of our country's Civil War. He maintained hope in an apparently hopeless situation. I felt the same way about children and single parents. I looked back at raising my own children and I still didn't know how I did it. It was a marathon each day, getting them off to school, picking them up when they were ill, cleaning up after them, waiting for them when they were out, worrying for them when they didn't have a clue — being a dad, a mom, and a grandparent, all at the same time.

Still, Lincoln made it through his war. I had made it through the day-to-day marathons, and I would make it through my Run. I realized how *easy* I had it. Lincoln did it daily for four years. My Run would only be for seventy-five days. I had only 43 days to go.

It was a wonderful day and I was twenty-six miles closer to Atlanta.

Day 33
Route: Springfield and on the road.
Weather: Sunny and warm
　Comment: The media is all over us. I feel my body breaking down.

DAY 33: MONDAY, JUNE 3

The sun was out all day again; this made three days in a row. I no longer had to run bundled up in layers of clothes. I could travel in shorts and either a T-shirt or, depending on how frisky I felt, an "I" shirt. Sunshine. No more wet. Hallelujah!

I told myself we needed to be like the plants and crops in the field; we needed to do more than just be warmed by the sun. We needed to grow as well. We needed to be our own crop, watering and feeding ourselves, taking care of the ground, doing everything necessary to achieve the harvest in mind: completing seventy-five marathons in seventy-five consecutive days.

Although many truck and car drivers were starting to identify us, we still needed to tell our story and get the word out. Springfield was a beautiful city, and everywhere we stopped people welcomed us. WQQI, WMAY, WNNS, WQLZ, WCVS, WSMI, WTAX, and WDBR were on hand to talk during our stay. We ended the day at the local Holiday Inn. These folks had certainly become good friends and Chris and I fell asleep happily, knowing the next day we would head toward Jacksonville.

Day 34
Route: On toward New Berlin and then Jacksonville, Ill.
Weather: Continued warm
  Comment: Angry drivers get in our way, but we move forward.

DAY 34: TUESDAY, JUNE 4

Chris and I left bright and early to get on the highway before the traffic was too heavy. I felt sad leaving Springfield. Everyone we had met was great. NBC was very supportive and said they would send their affiliates the tapes of me running down the highway, as well as the interview in front of Lincoln's tomb. We needed to continue sharing our story with those who would listen and, given the grassroots nature of the entire effort, the help from NBC was greatly appreciated. The effort could only continue to grow if the story was spread constantly and the message shared. I hoped, as the years came and went, we would have other events such as this and build upon those earlier successes. For now, though, we focused on the task at hand.

I had to dodge trucks and cars again all day and had another close call. This time, a blue van decided that I shouldn't be running on the highway or even the shoulder of the road. The driver must have thought the shoulder is reserved for motorized vehicles. I looked up just in time. I supposed in a way I was imposing on the cars' turf, but it still made me angry when drivers pointed their vehicles at me and cut away just before hitting me. Go figure.

Day 35
Route: Jacksonville to Greenfield, Ill.
Weather: Warm and getting hotter
   Comment: Chris and I fantasize of good food, a warm bed, and friends to laugh with.

DAY 35: SUNDAY, JUNE 5

As Chris and I headed toward Greenfield, Illinois, we traveled along a narrow and dangerous highway without shoulders. We could not keep from laughing though because it was no longer rain, rain, rain and its attendant chill, but rather sun, sun, sun and its attendant warmth.

The warmth of the sun was wonderful. However, the sun can also be unmerciful with its heat. To my dismay, I discovered it can burn even in hazy weather. Even though I used sun block, I ended up with severe sunburn. Still, it beat shivering in the wet and cold. I was so eager to feel the warmth of the sun after a month of being cold and wet that I foolishly ran without a shirt. (Do we not continue, even in our fifties, to sometimes see ourselves as we were at age nineteen?) Chris warned me about getting sunburned but I told him I needed the warmth. It was forever since we had seen sunshine. The entire month of May had been nothing but pounding rain and cold winds.

Although the heat felt good, it was also very draining. I desperately needed rest. Chris went to nearby stores to buy supplies so I had liquids and food, and he tried to provide opportunities for me to rest and be comfortable. But without the trailer or even a back seat, I had to rest sitting up in the front seat of the car. To add insult to injury, the air conditioning usually didn't work, and when it did function it didn't do so very well. Still, I sat, I rested, and it was warm on the road. I smiled and continued.

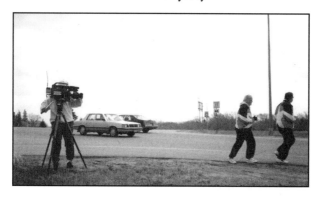

For a while Michael Durant followed along as our cameraman filming me as I ran. My friend Perry Williams joined me for a few miles while Michael asked me questions as he filmed. I answered his questions. He asked me how I felt. It was great to have the record of our Run on tape.

I answered, *"Each week differs. This morning I am out of breath. Put too much into days earlier in the week. We did 114 miles the past three days, running an average of thirty-eight miles each day. I have gone thirty miles today, so far. But as I run it improves. Maybe it's the sunshine. The day before the road was less safe. I felt like I was playing dodge ball with trucks. With the sun shining after a month of rain it just feels so good to be out here."*

At moments like that I reveled at how glorious it felt, running in the sun! I imagined I was both a conductor and the orchestra, my mind directing as my body played all of the instruments. The rhythm was incredible. Only someone in the groove of what they are doing would understand. From athletes to seamstresses to mothers rocking their babies and softly singing lullabies, all must know how I felt.

Maybe what made me feel better was the realization that not only was I continuing, but that a lot of media had picked us up and carried our story along the way. I was also heartened by the number of people who wanted to talk to Chris and me as we passed through their towns. This meant the story was getting out, that the Run was working, and that people were showing understanding. The question was: would it have staying power? Were we just another crusade of the month, only to be pushed off by the next? Doing this during the Olympics and Olympic Torch Run was supposed to help us. But at this point I wasn't sure it wasn't hurting us, as the very size of the Olympics was overshadowing everything else at the national level, including our Run. The thought was to ride on the wave of interest generated by the Olympics for people who overcome the odds, to go on and achieve great physical and mental feats, but the reality might be that the wave cleared everything else in its path.

In the past four weeks only one person had challenged me with the assertion that some single parents are single parents by choice, implying that, therefore, these parents deserve no support from their communities. But most single parents, I among them, are forced into that status by circumstance, not choice. Even when there are choices to be made, they are seldom easy ones. For example, I could have left my children to be raised by some more appropriate or ideal family – many told me I should – but I doubt very much that my children losing me after losing their mother would have accomplished much except to compound their feelings of abandonment and loss. They needed me, imperfect as I was, more at that time than ever.

Regardless of your position in this debate, the key point is not whether the situation is voluntary or involuntary, but that none of the children chose to be in single-parent families. The children still suffer in missing a parent. The children still suffer by losing precious hours with the single parent because that parent has an increased workload at home and may have to work a second job. *The children still suffer* with the friends who go away as well as those who treat them differently. *The children still suffer* the ordeal of having to work through the loneliness and a sense of abandonment. *The children still suffer* the false guilt, believing that somehow it is their fault. *The children still suffer* all the attendant emotional wounds to their sense of self-confidence and sense of worth. *The children* who are not the same gender as the single parent they live with *still suffer* the lack of a role model – consider that eighty percent of men in prison had no father or father figure in their lives as they grew up.

This Run held a serious purpose. But I also made people laugh, often without trying. People asked why I kept pulling up my shorts. I guess I looked funny doing so. The answer was simple: I was losing weight, which was a wonderful side benefit of running. I lost weight during my training. I lost even more on the Run. During training I dropped thirty-three pounds, going from 220 to 187. I started the Run weighing 187 pounds, and lost another twelve during the first month.

Despite my early euphoria, I was beginning to feel more poignant loneliness and physical discomfort. After thirty-four days I focused only on the highway now, looking ahead only a few feet or a few hours. To make decisions about where to stay or where to buy food was a major undertaking and simply beyond me. I was over the edge and like an army on the advance I had to rely on my logistics man, Chris, to handle the supplies and provide support. I had to keep my focus and save my strength. Chris rose to meet this very important occasion in his dad's life. I might be the man of the Marathon Run but Chris was very definitely the man of the hour.

At the end of the day I had an upset stomach. My body reacted differently on different days to all the pounding. Because Greenfield had no campground or Holiday Inns, Chris suggested that we go back down the road and stay at the same Holiday Inn again. We did. We were welcomed again. Thank you, thank you, and thank you, Holiday Inn.

Day 36
Route: Greenfield to Brighton, Ill.
Weather: Hot
   Comment: I begin to have mood swings. I need a hug.

DAY 36: THURSDAY, JUNE 6

My objective today was to arrive safely at Brighton, Illinois. Again, the shoulders on the side of the highway were narrow but thankfully traffic was light. My knees were very sore today and I wanted to rest my legs as much as possible. My sunburn was still bad, so I wore long pants and long sleeves to protect myself. The pendulum on my mood was swinging again. I really couldn't travel very far, only what we had planned. I felt quite sick. My mind was beginning to wander and I couldn't concentrate for long. It was hard for me to remember what I did yesterday, and again, I questioned why I was doing this to my body. If it weren't for my daily notes I realized I probably would remember little about the Run.

Because of the pain and my inability to focus I moved down the highway with an empty feeling. Only my son's positive comments or the smile of someone on the side of the road kept me going. Regular phone calls from Perry, Greg, J. Marie and others helped me find enough strength to continue. On this particular Thursday they sent verbal hugs; they made me smile. With continuing support from them, Chris and I still expected to make Atlanta by the middle of July.

Perhaps someone will make this kind of endurance trek an Olympic event, I mused. *Probably not. How was I doing this?* Just like my earlier life as a single dad, I knew why but I wasn't sure I knew how. Surely there must be an easier way but I was too busy pursuing this way to find it.

I couldn't get the plight of the parents – the single parents – out of my mind. I couldn't let them down; I couldn't let my kids down. Being a parent is like running a marathon every day, but for the single parent the run is longer, harder, and lonelier. Someone had to tell everyone that there are over 35-million people running these marathons every day, people who faced enormous obstacles as well as physical and emotional demands similar to those I faced each day on this Run. Damage control for them, as for me, came from their sleep, their faith, and their friends. But they needed more. They needed to know they weren't alone. They needed the love and support of their communities.

Day 37
Route: Brighton to Bunker Hill, Ill.
Weather: More hot weather rolling in
Comment: I feel my ability to stay focused dissipate. Chris takes over much of the media interviews.

DAY 37: FRIDAY, JUNE 7

I did a radio show today that gave me motivation to move forward. Some days everything just clicks. I was told you could hear that my heart was obviously into my commitment toward single parents and their kids. I continued to thank all the team members at every opportunity for their support, love, and dedication. They believed in me and in this cause.

On the radio show I recalled how my trainer, Scott Meier, had gotten me ready for this madness when others said it was not humanly possible. That no one had done it before meant nothing to Scott. My heart and desire to set goals and achieve them meant everything.

I was always amazed at how most people dismissed the idea at first, stating that neither I nor anyone else could do this to his body and survive to tell the story. The seemingly insurmountable issue was lack of rest. My age certainly was a factor, not to mention my heart attack a year prior. I have always felt I could do anything if I set my mind to it, but the Run so far had been a stretch. I had never run a marathon, much less two thousand miles. How foolish. No, crazy! I remembered Zak Manuszak, my business partner, helping me to understand what happens to your body when you push it. The information wasn't pretty. For an engineer, he seemed very knowledgeable about running and was helpful integrating this information into this dream of mine. He gave me the recipes for survival and achieving this feat. If I avoided the errors of others and paid strict attention to the signals of my body I could do it. Well, maybe.

As I persevered and trained and stayed with it people began to believe. And once they did, they didn't want to disbelieve. That a guy my age could do this made them all feel healthier and better. It seemed like madness, but I would make it. I had to.

Chris began answering more questions from the media and maturing right before my eyes, much to his and my delight. I was so thankful that he was there to experience the Run in person rather than hearing about it later, after the fact, and that he could learn and gain from the experience on his own.

Day 38
Route: Bunker Hill to Alton, Ill.
Weather: Hot
Comment: The media continues to be a friend. Chris questions how we made it this far. I question it too.

DAY 38: SATURDAY, JUNE 8

Saturday was a very long day. I covered more miles than I cared to count and ended in Alton, Illinois. As I ran into Alton two elderly women joined me and jogged alongside through the town. It had started to rain and both had their rain gear on as well as their oversized boots. They were sisters and both must have been well over seventy-five years old. They told me about their lives and how single parents had been looked down upon as they were growing up. Both ended up single parents themselves and had to work very hard to raise their families. As we continued together I felt myself become energized. We jogged slowly down the main streets of Alton, enjoying our conversation. WBTZ-TV met and interviewed all three of us.

My legs were sore. I had some recent trouble sleeping despite the luxury of the hotel rooms; the wear and tear of the ordeal was showing on my body. I found myself pushing hard to get to that next corner. I hoped I had enough of whatever was needed to get to tomorrow and then get through it.

Still, I knew that for someone who didn't really spend a great deal of time lifting weights, I was pretty strong. My strength to push forward was sometimes unbelievable. June 8th was a good reminder that strength is more than muscle. It is also attitude and mood.

Day 39
Route: Alton to East St. Louis, Missouri.
Weather: Warm and sunny
   Comment: NBC follows us all day. After my run, I can't even walk very well.

DAY 39: SUNDAY, JUNE 9

J. Marie, Michael Durant, and Mitch White drove more than thirteen hours from the Twin Cities to help with the media in St. Louis and to introduce the Run to the city. They brought me a teddy bear that looked like it got into some honey and had bumblebees sitting on its paws and face. It was a great gift, completely unexpected, and just the right thing to make me laugh.

KMOV-TV, KPLR-TV and KNLC-TV spent much of the day with me, capturing the grind. I tried to hide how bad my legs felt and how painfully my body was reacting. This was the most pain I had experienced for some time. It hurt just to step up onto a curb or step off. After taking his shots, Michael sent his video to the Twin Cities NBC affiliate, KARE 11, for their use. Once again, I was pleased to see the word getting out.

While we traveled the streets of St. Louis, especially East St. Louis, the presence of many single parents with their kids was evident. We were told later that no one runs in East St. Louis and comes out in one piece. How can that be? What are they afraid of? Everyone was friendly to us. Perhaps it's a lesson in life. If you are fair and open – real – others will treat you the same way. This daily marathon was like life. You care; they care. You help; they help.

I was asked why I was running to Atlanta rather than another city. I offered two reasons. The first was the presence of the Olympics there and my hope to use the timing to draw more attention to the plight of kids. The other reason was that I used to live in Atlanta, where I worked for The Coca-Cola Company. Two of my three children were born there.

I met with St. Louis City Councilman Francis Sleigh. We discussed children and their future and how the future of any city is dependent upon the future of its kids. We discussed day care and schools. We discussed the need for a federal department dealing with children, for a National Secretary for Children. We discussed the specific difficulty of being male and a single parent. Males of my generation were raised to be breadwinners. Even some women, who spout feminist rhetoric about wanting caring, sensitive men who can also do housework and help raise the children, are actually suspicious of any man who is primarily a caregiver, as if, in some way, he is no longer a real man. We talked about how we started out with a seven-member road crew, and how a combination of bad weather, mechanical breakdown, and other factors reduced that group to just Chris and me. We discussed the emotional help people had provided, which Councilman Sleigh attributed at least in part to the fact that people are indeed becoming much more aware that children are our future.

Day 40
Route: East St. Louis and south.
Weather: Hot and humid
  Comment: I'm just trying to keep my body from giving up.

DAY 40: MONDAY, JUNE 10

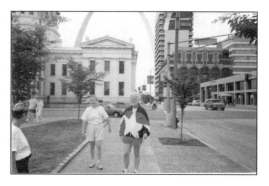

On the fortieth day of the Run, I was grateful for some special company: J. Marie had joined me now for the second day – most of the way through St. Louis, with a stop at the St. Louis Arch. I could never thank J. Marie enough for her support and help. She and her company provided many hours of free public relations. She put together media packets, many times working into the night to make certain we had enough for the next day or so. She always told the team members and me that public relations would be the thread that would gather the interest in what I was attempting to do. J. Marie was an excellent runner and although she claimed she could only go short distances she certainly did well and helped keep me going. Michael videotaped my efforts and would continue to capture much of my journey south, finishing his work in Atlanta. He wanted to produce what he expected to be an exciting documentary film of the Run. I couldn't wait to see it.

"The World of Sports is my world. I have seen first hand how individuals can accomplish the most difficult of challenges. In that same category is Terry's Run to Atlanta. Terry's Run was a 'World Series' event in itself ... and Terry and his son Chris did it for all the right reasons – to give back and to make a difference in the lives of our children and their families."

—Herb Carneal

The longtime voice of the Minnesota Twins and a National Baseball Hall of Fame member.

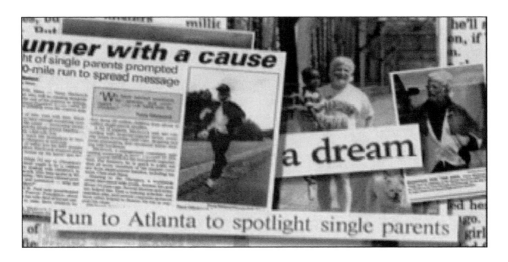

CHAPTER 14

DAYS 41 THROUGH 50

Day 41
Route: Still heading south from St. Louis.
Weather: High humidity
Comment: I was almost hit by lightening this afternoon in foolishly trying to outrun a big storm.

DAY 41: TUESDAY, JUNE 11

On Tuesday we visited the St. Louis United Way Day Care Center. Chris and I spent a couple of hours with a group of three-and four-year-old kids. Each child traced an outline of his or her hand and signed the outlines with Chris's help. It was really fun. We also went to City Hall and met with the president of the Aldermen Board and left our names with the Mayor's Office. At both places we continued to share our vision, to answer questions, and to tell some of the many stories we had accumulated on the Run so far.

I also spoke to a chapter of the Optimist's Club where Chris and I were warmly received. The members asked many questions and we could feel their strong support. It was becoming apparent that speaking and sharing stories about the Run was having an exciting impact. The Optimists knew about the Run before we arrived, having been notified of our route by a chapter we had previously visited; they wanted to help. They promised to notify other clubs along the way and to assist with the media in any way they could.

Although I was busy with my daily run, I also worked with Michael to finish up another part of the documentary. Michael wanted additional video shots of me warming up near the Arch, so I reluctantly went with him. He planned to pick up on our progress again when he rejoined us in Nashville, Tennessee. I just wanted to rest my sore legs, to rest my entire body, but I knew I must keep pushing ahead.

It was wonderful for our effort that the media was so active in St. Louis. In each town or city our stories and our accomplishments were creating strong interest. Two newspapers located Chris and me as we traveled the highway. It was clear to me at that point that the media and their interest were finally keeping up with us. Chris and I and the volunteers back home no longer had to try desperately to create interest and excitement as we went through each town. We had shown we could go this far. Now everyone wanted to see if we could go the rest of the way. The media cheered us on. They were becoming tellers of our story. We saw them on the highway waiting for us all the time. We were news – good news! Our credibility was real and this trek to Atlanta was drawing solid attention. We would do it. With Chris as my co-pilot, the rest of the crew in the Twin Cities supporting me, and with God's strength, of course we would do it!

This was the hottest day so far with the humidity well above ninety percent. Late in the afternoon, a huge thunderstorm engulfed us with heavy rain and lightning strikes. I almost made a serious mistake when I tried to out-race the storm. The rain followed me as I pushed forward down the highway and the lightning struck closer and closer. Chris helped me and I just made it to the car before the lightning came crashing down around us. We made our twenty-seven miles as planned, but it was a challenge. Being

Chicago Bulls fans, it didn't break our hearts to have to return to the hotel that night, where we watched the fourth game between the Bulls and the Seattle Supersonics, complete with unique lightning from Michael Jordan.

Day 42
Route: Toward Belleville, Ill.
Weather: Continued hot and humid
  Comment: Chris and I are hit by depression.

DAY 42: WEDNESDAY, JUNE 12

Most of the day's Run was on a narrow and busy highway. If that weren't challenging enough, the weather flip-flopped again from high heat and humidity to heavy rain and thunder. Chris and I took a couple hours off to buy an adapter so that our cell phone could be plugged into the car's lighter. Chris used the cell phone constantly, and the normal batteries we had been using just could not keep up with the demands.

At noon, I spoke to the Optimist's Club in St. Charles, Missouri. During the next five or six days, I would be running through sparsely populated countryside, so there were few opportunities to talk with many people. Also, since the next few days would offer few places to stay, we would have to backtrack after each day's Run to find a place to sleep. Even state parks were booked. We were all the more thankful for the letter from Holiday Inn.

It was good to know we were more than halfway through our journey to Atlanta. My body ached constantly and Chris was beginning to feel his own pain and depression. We made a fine team, both of us depressed and in pain. I hoped we could see it through as I continued running south toward Belleville and Carbondale, Illinois, looking forward to Kentucky.

> Day 43
> Route: Belleville to east of Nashville, Ill.
> Weather: Hot
> Comment: Chris works on inventory to keep us in water and bananas. I survived the cold and rain, but the heat is making it difficult to run.

DAY 43: THURSDAY, JUNE 13

Chris and I hit the highway early. We planned to put in as many miles as possible, forcing a one-day surge. *The Bellevue Democratic, Nashville News, Belleville Journal, Freeburg* and *The Spotlight* followed us and asked a lot of questions. Chris conducted his first lengthy radio interview with a phone interviewer from a station in Kentucky. I was very proud of him. He handled himself well.

Chris was working hard on nutrition, public relations, and navigation – making certain I was on the right road, going in the right direction – while also getting to his own appointments on time. Once again, I reflected that my son had matured right before my eyes.

> Day 44
> Route: Nashville to Du Quoin, Ill.
> Weather: Heat alerts and high humidity
> Comment: Emotionally, this is the worst day of the Run. I'm depressed. Have I hit the "second wall"?

DAY 44: FRIDAY, JUNE 14

Two days before Father's Day, the weather was hot again. High temperatures hit the mid-nineties with nearly one hundred percent humidity. Chris and I joined a Little League baseball game, umpiring one inning. He umpired first base and I put on the equipment and went behind the plate. It was fun and all the kids crowded around Chris and me after the game asking questions about the Run. When they asked us why we were doing it, it gave us another opportunity to talk about what it is like to be in a single-parent family and how this marathon Run symbolized the marathons that people run every day.

Chris and I were welcomed in Du Quoin, Illinois, by the Evening Call newspaper and WKYX-FM. They spent a considerable amount of time talking about MegaMarathon '96 with us and were supportive of what we are attempting to accomplish. During the afternoon I called WCCO radio in the Twin Cities and had my at least once a week chat with John Williams. John, who had been a solid supporter and continued to tell our story on the home front, said that I sounded down and depressed. I guess I was. The incredible pounding my body was taking would make anyone feel depressed. My emotional level rose and fell each day as the pain steadily became more intense. The past month and a half had really taken a toll.

Although I managed to get some wonderful rest, experiencing the deep sleep needed for healing each day, my mind obsessed on what Dr. Roth shared with me before I left about "the second wall." *Runners talk about it but few if any have actually experienced it.* It haunted me throughout the Run, like waiting for the other shoe to drop. I knew about the wall that a runner meets at about twenty miles during a single marathon, feeling that it's impossible to go on. But no one really knew much about the second wall. I had wondered as I ran each day what the second wall was like, whether I would hit it, and what I would experience if I did.

When it happened, I was totally unprepared. I was running down a highway in the bright sunlight and enjoying the warm breezes caressing my face. Suddenly, for no apparent reason, I started to cry, to sob uncontrollably. I wasn't really in pain. I was running well and feeling pretty good. I was just crying by the side of the road and had no idea why. All of a sudden I felt as though I had sunk into a black abyss. Depression. Loneliness. All-consuming. That's what John Williams noticed in my voice.

THE SECOND WALL

Was Chris having similar feelings? Each night he went straight to bed as soon as we found a hotel room. I might hide in a movie theater or soak in the hotel's pool. The last four weeks had been terrible for both of us. We were together, yet alone; alone, yet together. During the much needed phone contact some of our friends even said they were afraid for us.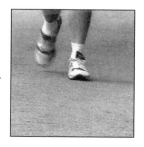

The loneliness was the worst aspect. The highways often were not friendly. The romance of the Run had long since departed. Cars and trucks continued to come too close to me as I dodged and worked my way past traffic. Chris could only helplessly watch and wince.

Still, we were blessed with enough rays of hope to get through each depression. We stayed in Du Quoin, Illinois, at Francie's Bed and Breakfast Inn – another complimentary and appreciated gift. This beautiful place was steeped in history and comfort. During the early 1900s Francie's housed hundreds of homeless children. Its founder was Martin Van Arsdale, also founder of the Children's Home & Aid Society of Illinois. What a perfect place to stay for a night of the Run.

Still, I felt so inexplicably sad. It had to be the second wall. I was depressed, lonely, and in need of hugs and good thoughts. I couldn't adequately explain how I felt, either on paper or verbally. It was truly awful. But I was still able to appreciate beauty and retain a sense of humor of sorts. That's good, I guess.

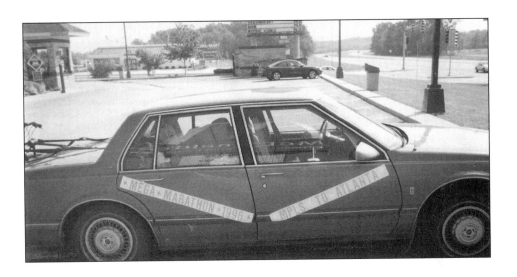

Day 45
Route: Du Quoin to Carbondale, Ill.
Weather: Temperature passes 100 degrees
 Comment: Kids run with me. It's a fun day. I feel my body is breaking down.

DAY 45: SATURDAY, JUNE 15

Chris and I took time after our normal run to do basic maintenance: wash dirty clothes, put a mailing together for all our friends, and see how we could repair the shock absorbers on our car. The car repairs would cost $450. Too much. It still wasn't as bumpy as the wooden-wheeled, no-shock Conestoga wagons of the pioneers. They would think we were traveling in luxury, and with that in mind we continued traveling.

We also had an opportunity to make a little boy's day. His name was Sam, and although he was in a wheelchair, he wanted to someday be a runner. I told him that if he believed, then someday he could. He really wanted a pair of my shoes so I took off the pair I had on and gave them to him along with one of my T-shirts. They were both far too large for him, but he promised me he would grow into them and would meet me on the highway someday.

I said I would welcome that day and join him any time he wanted. Sam and I hugged and then Chris and I had to leave.

Day 46
Route: Carbondale to Anna, Ill.
Weather: Temperature over 100, again.
Comment: Television stations follow us and film Father's Day segments. It's almost too hot to run and there is no place to hide from the sun.

DAY 46: SUNDAY, JUNE 16

It was the strangest Father's Day I had ever experienced. I had such mixed feelings facing the day: what father could have better (or worse) days than I was experiencing with Chris? Chris saw that I was fed every morning. He was always there. I really wouldn't have wanted his job. I sometimes wondered how he did it. So many times I saw him holding a phone in one hand and making my nutritious drink with the other, or searching for bananas for me to eat in order to keep the leg cramps at bay. Then he would hang up the phone, tell me what the local media wanted, made certain I had everything I needed and then drive off, saying he would meet me two or three miles down the road. You can't beat that.

We visited the First Presbyterian Church of Carbondale. Nearly everyone in church knew about the Run and welcomed us. After church, Chris and I met with WPSD-TV and WKPD-TV from Paducah, Kentucky. They wanted to put together a film for a special Father's Day broadcast, to be shown both that day and the following Monday night. We also found a touch football game. We joined everyone in the park and had a great time. We needed it, as our bodies and especially our minds were very sore and tired. Being with a group of people, having fun, and laughing seemed to be the best medicine for us.

I planned to leave about 8:30 a.m. in the morning the next day. Two television stations were scheduled to meet me on the highway. The NBC TV affiliate in Paducah planned to do another story on Chris and me.

Thus, despite the aches, pains, and the constant mental and emotional fatigue, it was one of the best Father's Days a dad could ask for.

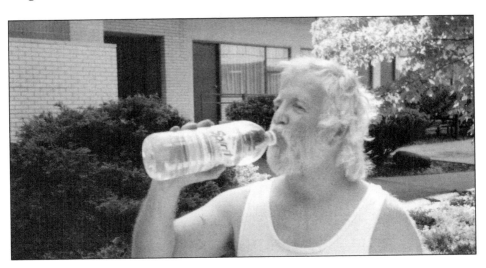

Day 47
Route: Anna to West Vienna, Ill.
Weather: Very hot and sunny.
 Comment: Steep terrain today. Chris and I question our sanity.

DAY 47: MONDAY, JUNE 17

Hot and sunny today – no surprise. What was once a world of cold and rain had become a world of eternal sunshine. It was also the beginning of some steep, hilly terrain. We started our day traveling toward Grantsburg, Illinois, and Paducah, Kentucky. This leg of the Run was a three-day trip through some big hills. In total, we planned to cover ninety-two miles and run through temperatures averaging 96 degrees with very high humidity. Had I craved the sun during those first few weeks? Be careful what you wish for!

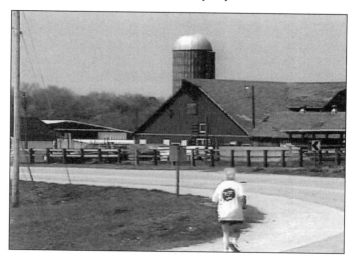

Day 48
Route: West Vienna to Reevesville, Ill.
Weather: Another heat alert
  Comment: My body is hurting terribly.

DAY 48: TUESDAY, JUNE 18

Traveling along the highway we saw few towns or people to talk to. Sometimes the noise of the traffic – swoosh, swoosh – as the cars and trucks rushed by unsettled me. I often felt curiously threatened as the whining trucks bore down on me. Dodging traffic didn't seem much like a humorous game anymore as it did earlier in my Run.

I also had stomach and chest pains, which I found more irritating than frightening. Chris took me to a local area hospital; the medical staff strongly suggested that I stay overnight because they thought I might have a heart problem. But I didn't want to.

I called J. Marie from the hospital around 11 p.m. to let her know. She wasn't surprised by the late call, having grown accustomed to our schedules and activities. This was yet another sign of support and acceptance – she was very open to being available at any hour, day or night, to provide us emotional strength if we needed it. I didn't want to alarm her, but I thought she would want to know about the hospital visit. She said when she picked up the phone on this call she knew something was wrong. I told her I had started to feel the pain in my stomach shortly after dinner and thought maybe it was just gas or something, but knew, given my history, that I should have it checked.

When I told her, she burst into tears. At first she thought I should quit. I almost agreed with her. She helped me work through the difficult decision whether to continue or give up. I knew when the discussion was over that I would keep going.

In the end, I stayed at the hospital overnight. Chris traveled back to Carbondale to sleep at the Holiday Inn. It was preferable to a night in a hospital bed. I made a deal with the doctors that unless they found something life threatening, I was going to leave by 9 a.m.

In the morning the doctors said their best guess was that my distress was probably caused by some fast food that I had eaten earlier in the day. What a relief. I was just happy it wasn't a heart attack. I was discharged at 9 a.m. and continued on my journey.

Day 49
Route: Reevesville to Brookport, Ill.
Weather: Hot, hot and humid
Comment: I struggle mentally with the trek. How long can I continue?

DAY 49: WEDNESDAY, JUNE 19

The sharp and almost indescribable pain that I experienced the first ten days of running had now matured into a dull ache. I consciously masked the physical damage I was inflicting daily upon my body. I hoped my body would heal itself as best it could.

I had read about men in prisoner of war camps and concentration camps. I learned that the key to their survival was attitude and a sense of optimism. I willed myself to use positive thoughts to counter the negative ones creeping out of the second wall's omnipresent depression. My reservoir of positive attitude and optimism had kept me from sinking to a point from which I couldn't come back. It was as if my whole life had been in preparation for this moment, in order to remain mentally fit for this great task. Positive attitude and optimism helped keep my body in a state of healing and renewal each day.

Even the most hardy, optimistic, and positive people experience the occasional dark night and wrenching soul-searching. The often-harsh nature of reality is a constant challenge to a positive outlook, an invitation to doubt. My mind could help heal my body, but my body could not heal my mind. My will and resolve also needed a rest. But when my mind began to rest, the doubts covered me like night clouds. Like Jacob wrestling with the angel, I was nearing the time when I would have to wrestle my own spirit. Would God carry me? The emotional toll on me, and also on Chris, continued to build. The second wall was certainly not yet behind us.

So, we did what we did best; we continued to cover more miles in a methodical fashion.

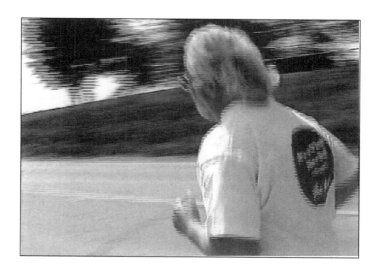

Day 50
Route: Brookport, crossing the Irvin Cobb Bridge, into Paducah, Kentucky.
Weather: Hot, what else.
Comment: We were the talk of Kentucky today. While crossing the bridge there was three miles of traffic behind me.

DAY 50: THURSDAY, JUNE 20

We entered Kentucky via the Irvin Cobb Bridge, which separates Brookport, Illinois, from Paducah, Kentucky. I was given a police escort as I ran across the two-mile-long bridge. The police later told me that we caused a record-setting traffic jam, backing up cars for more than three miles. Some of the people who passed us after we finished crossing the bridge gave a "thumbs up," others gave a salute with a different finger entirely. But that's life. Some people are proud to momentarily share your achievement; others see only how it inconveniences them.

"Having known Terry over twenty years, I never cease to be amazed by his dedication and commitment to the cause of improving the lot of children. This passion of Terry's was forever implanted in my mind during his "seventy-five marathons in seventy-five consecutive days," when he absolutely refused to quit in spite of lonely hours on deserted back roads, truckers who thought it was sport to aim at this solitary runner, and adverse conditions that would have caused most if not all of us to throw in the towel. Terry's dogged determination repeats itself in his refusal to back off his Foundation. Knowing it is a good, Terry has kept believing and driving to his goal of establishing the Foundation as the heart and voice of children everywhere."

—John Pope

President of John Pope Company

CHAPTER 15

DAYS 51 THROUGH 60

Day 51
Route: Paducah to Calvert City, Kentucky.
Weather: A break from the heat
Comment: I spent a few hours with kids and parents listening to their issues and sharing my ideas and support.

DAY 51: FRIDAY, JUNE 21

The most enjoyable part of talking with kids is that they are sincerely interested and have so many questions. We talked with kids at summer schools, in youth development programs, and everywhere else we found them. I promised to write to them if they first sent me their questions or comments.

Today, June 21st, after a few group discussion sessions were over, eight single parents, two of them men, joined me and we ran for about three miles together. Paducah, Kentucky is a great little city and it seemed that everyone knew about us as the nine of us ran through the streets with Chris leading the way in the car. I had fun with the impromptu parade and camaraderie. Later in the day I spoke to a group of kids in a group home. Again, they were full of questions. We also spoke to a large gathering at the Kentucky Dam about the Run and its grassroots nature. I was surprised and delighted to have people want to take pictures, referring to me as the "voice of the people." To give single parents and their children a voice was exactly the mission of the Run. Now we just had to hope someone was listening.

Day 52
Route: Calvert City, entering Land Between The Lakes national recreational area in Kentucky.
Weather: Mild weather continues
  Comment: How fast can bears run?

DAY 52: SATURDAY, JUNE 22

While running down a particularly deserted part of the highway, on this particularly beautiful day, I came across a black bear. A big bear. The bear was just stepping out of the woods and making all sorts of noises, breaking off small branches as it came right at me. We were face to face, staring at each other. I didn't know what to do. Fortunately, neither did the bear.

We both bolted, running as fast as we could to get away from each other. All I could think to do was talk to my legs: legs, let's go, legs, let's go. Two panicked animals, we mindlessly continued running, but parallel to each other, for nearly 300 yards. I understand bears have poor eyesight but a keen sense of smell and hearing. It could probably smell me but couldn't tell how big I was. I probably seemed as big to it as it did to me. That 300-yard stretch seemed like forever. I believe the bear was the noisier runner. All I could hear was snapping twigs and the bear grunting loudly, and myself huffing and puffing softly. I wanted it to be over. The bear was sprinting, not pacing, and for whatever crazy reason, I sprinted too. I didn't want to run at the bear, obviously, but the alternative was a suicidal dash onto the highway.

Finally, the bear veered off to the left and ran back into the woods. I stopped, shaken and then, again, redeemed by the humor of it all, started to laugh. When Chris came driving back for my feeding, he found me exhausted, sitting on the side of the highway laughing. When I told him my story he roared with laughter and wished he had been here to film it.

After resting and catching my breath I continued on down the Kentucky road. As I set off, I noticed something that had become common throughout the Run: dogs, lots of dogs, most slumbering, some barking, some snarling, and, on occasion, a number of them harmonizing in quite a symphony of sound. Every time I came across a dog, I would think of Charlie. I sure missed him.

Day 53
Route: Continuing along the lonely road.
Weather: Warms up again to over 100 degrees
Comment: Media continues to follow us. It seems everyone is pulling for us.

DAY 53: SUNDAY, JUNE 23

This Sunday, along our path, people turned out *en masse* and ran with me for almost a mile. There must have been more than one hundred people – nearly everyone in the small town. I was heartened that people were really beginning to understand the seriousness of this trek and why all of us must do something to help this large and growing group of over thirty-five million people.

I was interviewed by The Tennessean newspaper for Tuesday's edition and we planned to meet with the paper again on Wednesday when we arrived in or near Nashville.

My good friend Dr. Roth called and helped me with my focus for the remaining three weeks. He seemed so wise and all knowing. As a runner, he understood and appreciated what I was going through emotionally, and he provided the strategies to retain my focus and to instill additional meaning into each day and hour.

After the Run, Chris and I made the long drive back to the same Paducah, Kentucky Holiday Inn to sleep, and to prepare for yet another day.

Day 54
Route: Leave Kentucky and head to Dover, Tenn.
Weather: Nearly unbearable heat
  Comment: Thanksgiving now has a new meaning following our turkey run.

DAY 54: MONDAY, JUNE 24

Chris and I left Kentucky and headed toward Dover, Tennessee. The weekend's heat wave hovered around us. It was the first time I experienced a heat wave alert. On Sunday afternoon the temperature had reached more than one hundred degrees and the humidity was nearly as high, making it difficult to run or even walk. Just prior to leaving the great State of Kentucky, as I was approaching the car for my rest and snack, Chris waved at me to turn around. I did, and what I saw was unbelievable.

Following behind me up the highway was a flock of wild turkeys. Chris called out to them that I wasn't their dad. But as I continued up the highway, so did they. They didn't seem to be afraid and kept about twenty feet behind me as I jogged. Finally they went into the woods as I neared the car. We had another great laugh.

As we were leaving Kentucky we encountered a river flowing softly, looking so inviting, and with a small embankment. Chris and I exchanged a quick look and without saying a word, we jumped right in. The coolness of the river was so refreshing in the unbearable heat. I found myself wishing there was a river we could follow all the way to Atlanta.

We left the rolling hills of Kentucky and entered the mountains of Tennessee. It was time to rethink the plan; because of the heat I had to consider running at different hours. I would probably leave much earlier each morning, take the mid-afternoon off, and finish up the day by running in the early evening.

> **Day 55 and 56**
> Route: Dover, through small towns, on our way to Nashville, Tenn.
> Weather: More heat
> Comment: Each step is more difficult. Individual supporters continue to surprise me.

DAY 55 & 56: TUESDAY & WEDNESDAY, JUNE 25-26

We traveled through several small towns of Tennessee on our way to Nashville. Michael joined us and filmed a few more days of my trek. His presence was a welcome change and another morale boost. While going through one of the small towns I was stopped by an elderly woman standing with her cane in front of her home. She said she had never been a single parent but that her daughter was and she wanted to help. She gave me a five-dollar bill. It looked like it had been folded and stuffed in a special hiding place for a long time. I thanked her and she smiled.

The temperature continued to hover in the high nineties. Fortunately, the air conditioning in the car was beginning to work a little. I'm not sure whom the heat would be worse for: me, running in it, or Chris, sitting in the hot car all day.

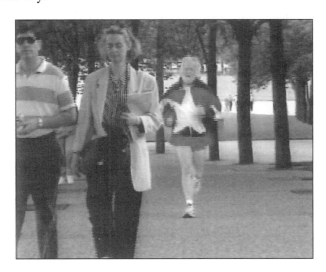

Day 57
Route: Enter into Centennial Park in Nashville, Tenn.
Weather: Lots of heat
Comment: Big crowd of 35,000 people. It sent me from heat exhaustion and near collapse to exhilaration.

DAY 57: THURSDAY, JUNE 27

As we reached within three miles of Centennial Park in Nashville the heat began seriously affecting me. I sat down next to the highway while Chris gave me water. I was scared. My health was diminishing fast. I was disoriented and overly warm, even with bottles of cold water emptied on my head and neck. I knew I was nearly done for the day and I hoped the feeling of panic would soon pass. After some rest I finished my run into Nashville.

As Chris and I entered Nashville we encountered a festive atmosphere. People in cars honked their horns and waved as Chris and I arrived at Centennial Park. The newspaper, *The Tennessean*, followed along and covered my arrival, as did Michael. As the sun set and the lights came on, the city sparkled and grew more festive. The Olympic torch was being carried through town. Although it was nighttime, the lights and the peoples' high spirits made it seem like midday. I even ran with the Olympic torchbearer! About thirty-five thousand people made their way to the park to celebrate our passing through town – the Olympic torchbearer, and me, a torchbearer of a different kind.

It was awesome to be in the midst of the Olympic torch's passage and to be a part of the celebration. Impressive as the torch entourage was, with the ambulances, the cars, and the many people milling around, it couldn't adequately express the meaning the torch held for me. I had been scheduled to carry the torch a couple of weeks earlier back in Minneapolis, but I couldn't, obviously, because I was already more than four hundred miles away, running. I wondered what we could do to whip up this kind of enthusiasm for the daily marathons of single parents and their children. I wouldn't always have the coattails of the Olympics to ride on, but the cause for which I was running would certainly outlast the summer games.

I talked to the media while Michael and Chris wandered through the park. I shared my story on two local radio stations. Chris and I also talked with members of the Striders Running Club of Nashville and left literature for everyone. All in all, it was a great day.

Day 58
Route: Through Nashville, heading south.
Weather: Warm, less humid.
   Comment: Betweens runs, I talked with many kids and families.

DAY 58: FRIDAY, JUNE 28

The day started with a special event held at Planet Hollywood in Nashville. We received marvelous hospitality from Planet Hollywood. It was fun talking with the Nashville manager and discussing Arnold Schwarzenegger's work for a cause dear to him: physical fitness. Indeed, I was told he just missed being able to join us at the beginning of the Run in the Twin Cities, a surprise my daughter Teri Sue tried to set up. It would have been a wonderful gift.

Sarah Smith, head of Oasis Crisis Center, told the assembled crowd that I was running to raise awareness of the services needed for single parents across the country. She noted that many in the crowd were struggling with single-parent issues, including a wide range of frustrations and challenges. She read a proclamation from Mayor Phil Bredesen declaring June 28 *Children Are Forever Day*. The proclamation was another example of how the hard work was beginning to pay off. *Someday*, I thought, *I will look back and know that my three months on the road and all the hard work of the many volunteers resulted in something very special.* I spoke briefly, feeling a bit like Forrest Gump. A TV reporter told me that *The Guinness Book of World Records* is three consecutive daily marathons. Somehow, until that day, the fact that I had shattered the record and was going for far more had completely escaped me.

Later in the afternoon, we visited the Oasis Crisis Center and spent a couple more hours talking with the kids and listening to their stories. WXIA-TV, WSB-TV, WGNX and WAGA were on hand to catch much of our time in their city. A large percentage of the kids at the Oasis Center are from single parent-homes; far too often they drop out of school and, in turn, become single parents themselves. They are part of the reason for the Children Are Forever Foundation, and one of the many things we hoped to help change.

Day 59
Route: Outside Nashville, heading to Murfreesboro, Tenn.
Weather: Unbearable heat returns
  Comment: My night was not restful.

DAY 59: SATURDAY, JUNE 29

We left Nashville, Tennessee, and headed toward Murfreesboro, where we were interviewed by the *Daily News Journal*. The temperature was in the high nineties. At this point we lost another valuable member of the team, as the car's air conditioning finally gave out.

Both of my ankles were really hurting. I wasn't surprised. After all, I had been running every day for eight weeks. Chris insisted that I go to the hospital emergency room for x-rays. The doctor asked that we look at the pictures together. I was surprised at what I saw. The doctor, in a serious tone, showed me fractures on each ankle and damage to my left kneecap. He strongly suggested that I rest and keep both ankles in an upraised position for the next ten days. Despite the x-rays, I'm not sure he fully comprehended what I had been through so far or what was yet ahead.

It was a tough call. My right ankle had a fracture and my right heal had a bone spur. My left ankle sported a hairline crack. I smiled. I said I would put them up after I got to Atlanta. I still had ten more miles that I wanted to cover that day.

Day 60
Route: Through Murfreesboro, south to Manchester, Tenn.
Weather: Hot and humid
   Comment: I would rather have the pain of the Run than the pain of the needles.

DAY 60: SUNDAY, JUNE 30

The dilemma of my ankles amounted to a mental exercise. I couldn't completely ignore the diagnosis of fractures in my ankles. I couldn't ignore the fact that the doctor wanted me to stay off my feet for ten days and avoid running during this time. Logically, I could not continue. I should not continue.

I continued anyway.

I appreciated the doctor's concern, but I had thought about the possibility of injury before the Run began. When I had my heart attack in the middle of my seventeen months of training I thought of all those who had it worse than I did. I thought of kids who had it worse than my kids, of two-parent and single-parent families working two and three jobs, of kids going to bed hungry, of kids not having a role model at home, of the many latch-key kids who had no one to greet them when they come home from school. They needed to know that others care, that others were rooting for them to succeed in life. There was so much hoopla at the Metrodome, so many interviews on radio, TV, and in newspapers. So many people were counting on me. How could I even consider not continuing?

The cliché, *no pain, no gain*, came to mind. So many people had done so much for me; I had to stick it out for two more weeks. When I compared my situation to that of others I realized that I had much to be thankful for, much to give back for what I had received. No amount of pain could stop me now. I would stop only if my body literally couldn't function. Too much was at stake. Too many children would benefit if we could get communities to see their plight and act on their behalf. The Finish Line was so near. Only two weeks to go. I had to go on.

"I was on Everest for seventy-five days and I'll tell you what – I would much rather go climb that frigid mountain one more time than attempt running seventy-five marathons in seventy-five consecutive days as you did, Terry. Congratulations on your feat of feet."

—Eric Alexander

Led blind climber up Everest in 2001

CHAPTER 16

DAYS 61 THROUGH 70

Day 61
Route: Through Manchester and into the foothills.
Weather: Slightly cooler today.
Comment: Met with old friends. Found out a close friend died, so I dedicate the Run's next few days to him.

DAY 61: MONDAY, JULY 1

While Chris and I rested from the heat, we prepared for the coming week. Both of us were thinking of the Tennessee Mountains ahead and the trouble they would cause for my knees and ankles, and for our car. We had put more than nine thousand miles on the car because of all the back and forth Chris had to do. The shocks were gone; the air conditioning was gone. We hoped the rest would simply hold up long enough to finish the Run. We had just two more weeks. Through Day 61, I had run about sixteen hundred miles. Not a bad ratio in comparison with the car.

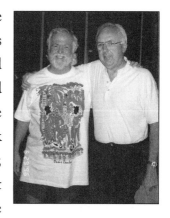

On Monday I saw a good friend, Dick Yutendale, and his lovely wife, Marie, whom I had not seen for many years. Chris and I had dinner at their home and enjoyed their company very much. Dick and I talked about old times and our life right out of college with General Motors. Dick was doing well. It felt good for both Chris and me to be able to relax and kick back after our daily trek. Thanks, Dick and Marie.

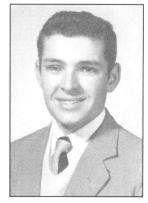

I also received word that one of my best friends, Melvin Monteith, had passed away. He and I went to school together in North Troy, Vermont. My Run the next day was dedicated to Mel.

Day 62
Route: Mountains in the distance.
Weather: Hot, less humid
Comment: Chris and I fantasize about our friends and even Charlie. Every hour we talk about quitting. It's difficult to stay focused.

DAY 62: TUESDAY, JULY 2

I discovered a renewed sense of urgency to finish the Run. So much time and preparation went into MegaMarathon '96, I began to feel as though completing it was my destiny. My latest mantra: *I must go on. Just under two weeks to go! Today is Melvin's day!*

Chris and I persevered toward Chattanooga, Tennessee. The weather remained as hot and humid as ever. For more than ten days the temperature was over ninety-five degrees and the humidity almost unbearable. I needed more liquid and more food in that kind of climate. Chris kept a tight schedule to manage the increased back-and-forth driving required to keep me hydrated and energized, while still attending to, well, everything else.

With the Fourth of July holiday coming up, Chris and I suffered another round of acute loneliness. We were concerned about where we would spend the holiday. This may seem a minor consideration but in our own world of the road, holidays and times of special meaning loomed with far more importance than at home. Our loneliness and confusion caused us more than ever to miss the friends who normally spent time with us, listened to us, and provided hugs and support. And we missed Charlie, who had gone back to Minnesota with the truck.

The journey was creating intense frustration for both of us. More and more often we each misinterpreted comments intended by the other to be encouraging, causing great emotional ups and downs. We were almost desperate for attention and motivation to continue. It was tough – the second wall was really tough to break through. I was never sure that I *had* broken through it or that I ever would. Chris may have, but more than sixty days into the Run, I certainly had not.

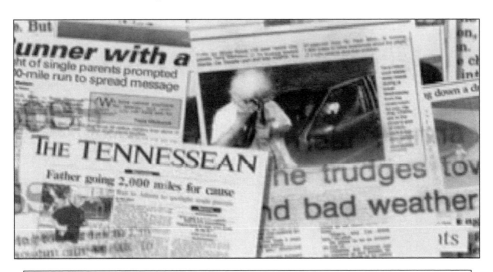

Day 63
Route: About 50 miles from Chattanooga.
Weather: Less humid and bearable
    Comment: I never met a mountain I couldn't climb. Actually, I almost lost.

DAY 63: WEDNESDAY, JULY 3

We entered southern Tennessee almost fifty miles from Chattanooga. There was virtually no shoulder along the entire route. The road wound around, and up and down, and around again in a seemingly endless coil as it hugged the mountains. It was a nightmare of blind corners and difficult terrain.

While I stretched, a truck driver stopped and asked if I needed help. I didn't, but it was certainly nice to be reminded that some people care. During the course of the Run people did stop several times to offer help. The local paper even invited us to a Fourth of July party. These offers were lifelines at times and particularly so on the Fourth of July.

Over the past two months we had stopped in every town or city we came to. I had spoken on Sundays in whatever church would have me, never missing a Sunday service. I had talked with children ranging from three-year-old toddlers to college-age students. Everyone wanted to ask questions to better understand why someone would do this. Kids and adults had waited along the road for me. Each day the number of people waiting for us to arrive had grown. Some people ran with me for a while. Running clubs along the route had joined in for short distances.

We had had many positive experiences speaking en route to Atlanta and most of those opportunities were due to the stories in the local papers. In those smaller towns and rural areas, the local newspapers were like the arteries of a giant community heart, carrying the lifeblood of information, connecting everyone. Throughout the Run we were grateful for every inch of type and every bit of publicity these publications contributed.

In the later stages of the Run when I needed a warm memory to boost my day, I reflected on a family I met in Iowa. I was running down a rural road one day and came upon a family waiting for me to arrive. They waved me down to join them. The father, mother, young daughter and young son just wanted to talk. I shared my experiences that day and they all hugged me and wished me good luck. The little girl gave me a gift before I left, a note I read many times as I traveled down unfamiliar and often frightening roads. She had written, "Thank you for doing this for kids who are not as lucky as I am. I have both my mommy and daddy."

There were plenty of other memories to pull me through that last week and a half. During the Run I visited many schools to talk about the Run and its purpose. I sat on floors, little chairs, rugs, sofas, and all kinds of things. I played games in the playground with children. I was always amazed at how eager they were to have me join their games and playtime. I ran high-five gauntlets of kids. They drew pictures of the Run and of their thoughts and feelings about being from single families. Shy first graders became loud and proud. My heart always went out to them and always will.

I was amazed and delighted by the many people, from all the organizations, who talked with us, reminding me of the unique community make-up of our country, of individuals joining others for the purpose of pursuing a wide range of interests and pursuits. I hoped some of these community associations might help more with the kids of single-parent families after our discussions of the Run and its purpose. It would be so wonderful if something more could be done to take care of the latchkey kids and help prepare them for their roles as citizens in their communities.

When Alexis de Tocqueville recorded his observations on American life in the mid-nineteenth century, he noted that one thing people in communities all across our nation had in common was the belief that they could solve problems without having to inherit money or be elected to public office. He saw this as a new dimension of democracy. Maybe we need to stress this important dimension of our democracy in the civics lessons in our schools, from K-12 through college. We need to remind ourselves that taking personal responsibility makes our communities what they are. Healthy communities make a healthy nation.

Many kids today have little positive exposure to the people in their community. Their most familiar community is an electronic one. National legislators seem to think that the only neighborhoods that count are the two on either side of the Capitol building in Washington, D.C., the neighborhoods of the Senate and the House. And yet the real assets of this country are not there, but in the neighborhoods of our cities

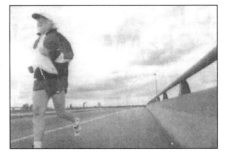

and towns and the farm communities of our rural areas. We, as a country, are only as strong as our local neighborhoods.

As I ran through community after community I realized that much of the democracy of this country appeared silent, under the radar, off the TV screen, outside the glare of political and cultural celebrities. Daily democracy may be out of the spotlight, beyond where correspondents and politicians spend their time, beyond that part of their lives which seems more and more to be endless fundraising, but it is there. As I think about the new millennium I wonder, will we find ourselves still a democracy fifty years from now?

We should not look for the answer in government or politics, but within ourselves. The answer will be determined by whether or not we, the people, claim and exercise our power as citizens. Too many national, state, and local governing bodies treat citizens as clients or recipients. Indeed, they use these actual terms! Some even refer to people as their customers. Unfortunately, this view too often forgets that these customers are also the board of directors. Even more unfortunately, the citizen/customers sometimes forget it themselves.

My Run through towns and villages and cities renewed my hope and faith in America.

Being a citizen is another daily marathon. I run into citizen marathons every day. We need to re-associate our identities with citizenship, not commerce. (Commercial values and identities are fine, but only in commerce). We need to identify ourselves as friends, neighbors, partners, and citizens. I run into people every day who live the vision of seeing life as a glass half-full, not half-empty. But unless they exercise their power as citizens they can just sit back while the suits, the paid professionals, take over their communities. These professionals keep harping on half-empty, as if to be positive would expose the truth that many of them, and their careers, are unnecessary for the survival of the communities in which they work.

Day 64
Route: Up the great Smokey Mountains.
Weather: Mild temperatures
Comment: Wow!

DAY 64: THURSDAY, JULY 4

Well rested, Chris and I covered what was probably the most difficult section of the route. Before the day ended, I ran up the great Smokey Mountains, a constant upward climb. Once at the top, I set off on the long, torturous trip down. The temperature hovered at ninety-seven degrees; very, very hot, even on the tree-lined roadways.

Climbing the winding mountain road was a real challenge logistically. Chris wasn't able to stop at two- or three-mile intervals and wait for me because he couldn't find a place to turn around. In order to provide me with liquid and food he had to make longer back-and-forth trips than usual. The uphill road was very winding and had no shoulder; that combined with a fair amount of traffic, made it difficult and dangerous to run. The constant push to go uphill and to still maintain my breath and strength became a real challenge. I have never tackled such a steep incline before (or since).

I had training and natural stubbornness on my side, but this would have been a real push for anyone's body. With each step I strained to keep my breath constant and slow. My calves bulged and craved for a break. It seemed the top would never come and I only kept going because of my faith in God, my faith in our cause, and the faith of all the people working for the Run back in the Twin Cities. Faith and friends were more important than ever. It had long been clear to me that without them I could not have made this trek. Thinking of kids, thinking of single parents is all well and good, but to overcome that level of pain, loneliness, depression, disorientation and lack of focus at the bottom of each hill, staring at the climb ahead, required something more transcendent than a cause. It required the unhesitating faith of loved ones.

I finally rounded the last corner to the top. If my knees had been able to scream, the sound would have been heard throughout the valleys below.

Instead, Chris cheered. He was sitting in the car at a lookout, which was his turn-around spot for much of the latter part of the mountain trek. He had been amusing himself with the video camera, doing a play-by-play description of me as I plodded up the mountain. He showed it to me and it was really very funny. He had a mantra only a son could make up and only a father could appreciate and enjoy: "Come on dad, you can do it! Little man, big mountain, little man, big mountain." As I watched the tape I broke up with laughter.

Most people might think that, having ascended to the summit, the hardest part was over. Not so. The hardest part was going downhill. Running downhill is far harder on the knees. Chris pleaded with me not to run or walk down the very steep, shoulder-less roads. He wanted me to ride in the car. But riding in the car even one mile had not been an option on this Run and would not be an option in the Smokey Mountains. I was determined to cover every mile with foot power only.

Along with the great pain in my ankles I was feeling quite nauseous as well, so I decided to ride Chris's bike down the mountain, with Chris driving the car behind me. I felt that this way I could make the descent in an ethical yet survivable manner. I rode the bike down the long, winding and steep road, down the other side of the mountain. It was a real adventure. Chris said at times I was going almost thirty miles per hour. Believe me, I hung on for dear life. There were a number of irritated drivers behind Chris. Because of the turns they couldn't pass, but because of those same turns Chris and I couldn't go any faster. It's not as though they were really being held up; they just thought they were. It must have looked crazy to them to see this guy going hell bent for leather on a bicycle down this steep and winding mountain. We made it. I was still in one piece. Total miles that day:

thirty-nine. Even with the bike ride, I had still run more than twenty-eight miles, putting one foot in front of the other.

Again Holiday Inn helped with a nice room. The next day, I planned to run into Chattanooga. My only thought as I closed my eyes and crossed my fingers was a desperate hope that we would find a Holiday Inn there as well.

After Chris fell asleep, I went to the hotel lobby to fax material to our PR firm, Nemer Fieger and Associates. While there, I was asked by a couple if I would consider playing Santa Claus during the upcoming holidays. They said the pay would be about $5,000. I said I would call them. This gig could be anywhere in the U.S. With my white beard some have said I look like their ideal Santa Claus.

Maybe that is what I was doing, running down the highways of this country playing Santa Claus. But my bag was empty. And instead of eight tiny reindeer I had ten tiny toes. But I sure wished I could be Santa to all kids.

Regardless, it certainly seemed strange to mix my holidays, discussing playing a Christmas Santa Claus and conjuring up images of snow and winter on that very hot Fourth of July.

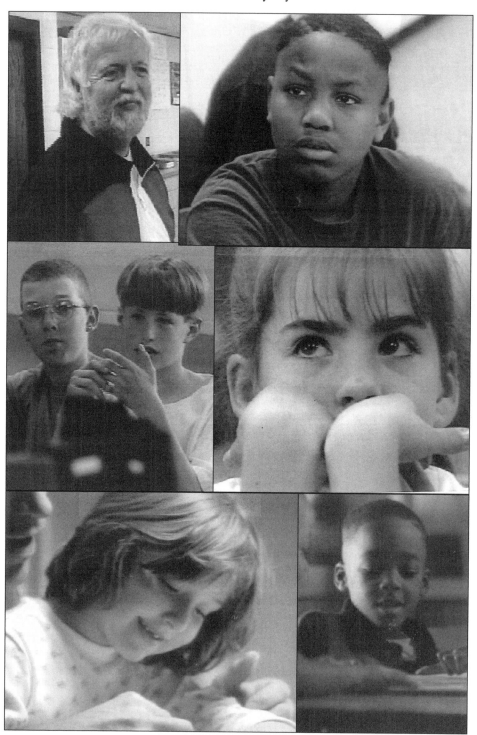

Day 65
Route: North of Chattanooga, Tenn.
Weather: Back to 100 degrees
  Comment: Crowds gather wherever we go. The story is out.

DAY 65: FRIDAY, JULY 5

Chris and I started the day early. As expected, the temperature again reached the low 90s. I began with a 15-mile jog to the center of Chattanooga. By starting early I was able to put in the necessary miles before a meeting scheduled for 10 a.m. Chris and I visited a day-care center, one of the many highlights of my trip. More than one hundred fifty children, in small groups of fifteen or twenty, listened to my message and asked wonderful questions. The children presented me with a special card, which I will always cherish. It was over six feet high and signed by everyone.

Next, we visited a large family center. Again, I talked with many single-parent family members. We ate lunch with the kids, answering their questions as I had at the day care center. The executive director said she would help in any way she could throughout the weekend to introduce Chris and me to the community and local media.

After finishing the day, I asked another Holiday Inn if they could help with a room. The innkeeper came through again and Chris and I had a place to rest and sleep. After running twelve more miles in the evening, I really needed to soak my feet. Although I had had no blisters thus far (which I attribute to the shoes and socks), my ankles were very pained and each chance I was given to use a hot tub or pool, I took. To this day I'm still saying, "Wow! Thanks again, Holiday Inn."

Day 66
Route: Enter Chattanooga.
Weather: Hot enough to cook an egg on the pavement. Honest!
Comment: We feel the presence of the finish line looming in Atlanta.
  Maybe we can do it!

DAY 66: SATURDAY, JULY 6

During a roadside television interview I was asked if the President of the United States was in front of me, what would I say to him? I thought about it for a moment and the answer was clear. I would say, "Mr. President, are our children the future of this country? If so, then why don't we have a National Secretary of Children, a Cabinet-level position?"

That comment hit the front pages of newspapers the entire week. I really believe that someday we will have a Secretary of Children. Why not? We must! As I ran I often wondered how it is that we can be less concerned about our kids than about defense, or the environment, or commerce, or labor, or the treasury, or education, or health, or housing. None of these subjects has children at its core. I can't help thinking that if the world evaluated every action on the basis of what is good for children, many of the terrible calamities caused by the childish acts of adults would end, especially domestic violence at home and armed conflict outside the home. When we have kids, we should start evaluating our actions based on how they affect our descendants for the next hundred years.

All in all, it was a great day. We continued on toward Marietta and Atlanta, Georgia, feeling excitement build with every step.

Day 67
Route: Continue through Chattanooga on way to Georgia.
Weather: Warm, but cloudy.
   Comment: Chris and I are sick. I feel like I can't go much further.

DAY 67: SUNDAY, JULY 7

Chris was very sick the previous night and stayed in bed for more than twelve hours. I was sick all day today, especially while running, and blamed the heat. Chris laughed and said it's what I was doing to my body each day that was making me sick – not just the heat.

Whatever the reason, both of us had been fighting sickness for about a week now, and the heat easily sapped most of our strength away. Chris said I look tired. I thought he was eating too little. He hadn't slept well either, but he continued to maintain a positive outlook for the most part. I had a slight fever to start off the week and hadn't kept my food down well for almost two days. I kept thinking I must have the flu and I kept telling myself that with one week to go no illness was going to derail me.

ABC, NBC and CBS filmed my Run and interviewed both Chris and me for their individual segments. Again, the media was great. Their belief in what we were trying to accomplish provided us with continuing strength and focus.

Day 68
Route: 190 miles to Atlanta.
Weather: Hot and sticky
Comment: We feel the emotional strain, but we believe that, somehow, we will get to Atlanta.

DAY 68: MONDAY, JULY 8

We were now about one hundred ninety miles or so from Atlanta. The temperature in Atlanta was 112 degrees. Even so, I looked forward to moving southward. We were about out of money again, so we couldn't spend much on anything but gas.

That afternoon, a farmer stopped me as I jogged past. He was sitting on his fence while his daughter and son moved bales of hay onto their truck. The farmer asked why I was doing this Run and he seemed really interested in the purpose. He said that he hadn't thought of the issues before now, but it made sense and that several of his friends were single parents. He said he never gave it a thought before, but there was a lot of pain in those families, and we should have everyone help out. He then thanked us for our effort.

We contacted the Christian Business Men's Committee (CBMC) and other organizations in Tennessee that day. We called friends in Atlanta to see if they could find rooms for us for the coming weekend. With the Summer Olympics in town, it seemed almost impossible to find a place in or near Atlanta.

We were a few days from Marietta, Georgia, where Chris and Jason were born. Chris noticed that I was very sore. He told me not to worry about it, that I can do it, that we are sixty-seven days down and only eight to go. I laughed. "That's easy for you to say," I told him. But sometimes I wondered who had the toughest job. All I had to do is run, write, and sleep. Chris had to coordinate and take care of everything else. If you wanted to get right down to it, it wasn't his Run. It was mine. Chris spent his whole time in a completely different world of serving. I had done that as a single parent because I was serving my kids. I wondered aloud if I could ever do for someone else what Chris was doing for me. Chris hooted and asked me about all the companies I had already done it for. I am all the more proud and delighted at the good-humored effort he made at what otherwise was not a very humorous occupation for him. And besides, I got paid for helping companies. Chris's external compensation came in gratitude only.

Michael rejoined us to film more of the Run. He wanted to interview me in a quiet place. Of all places, we wound up in a large shower stall. It reminded me of a story my friend Peter Jessen told me, about a book he read in college, *Memoirs of a Renaissance Pope*, by Pope Pius II. The Pope noted that the only place he could have a meeting without being overheard was in the privy. Peter used to joke about this when people whispered or tried to sound important or particularly severe. He would tell people that this is how the "Privy Council" was born, and that the meeting they were having was like meeting in an ancient privy. I used to laugh at the story. Now it was my turn to confer in the dubious dignity of the privy.

Michael asked me to share my thoughts as we came to the end of our time in Tennessee and prepared to cross the state line into Georgia and head on to Atlanta. He asked me how I was feeling. I wasn't sure anymore. I no longer knew how to answer that question. I could only ramble, which I did. I felt weird, almost as if I were moving and speaking in slow motion. During the interview, my head seemed to move slowly, as if it were not a part of my body. I sat slumped on a stool. I know I sounded strange.

I know this is the hardest thing I've ever done physically. My ankles really hurt. Those hairline fractures we saw in the x-rays aren't doing any better. I'm surprised that my knees feel pretty good, though. I have been really sick the last few days though. I can't keep food down Depression is raising its ugly head. I miss my friends and family. I miss my life. I am anxious to get to Atlanta and get this over with.

I think we are doing a lot of good, but I can't tell. I've done about as much as I can do with my body without more serious complications. I think what I've done is about as much as I ever want to put my body through. By today we have come over 1,800 miles. I'm anxious and moody. I miss all the little things in life we so take for granted, like eating, and sleeping, and sitting when you want to, and not moving when you don't want to, and reading the paper, and keeping up with events in the world. I'm irritable. I seem to be reading negatives into all the little things people say.

My mind plays games and tricks on me. I find I'm trying to remove myself from what is going on around me. I find it more and more difficult to find the right things to say. Sometimes it seems as if I am standing outside myself watching myself perform for the media, answering their questions. I cry easily about anything and everything. I feel so sad. I ramble. I will talk incessantly where I would normally quit. Chris isn't saying anything about it, but I must be driving him nuts. I wring my hands. I don't like pain yet there is constant pain at all times somewhere in my body. I haven't slept well for more than a week. I feel nauseous all the time.

I was physically, mentally and emotionally exhausted: *Every morning I'm relying on the people at home to get me back on the road. On the one hand, I am glad the Run is about over, but on the other hand, I wish it could continue because of the good that I sense is being accomplished. I am constantly thinking of things that I need to do. I am normally not sad, but I am sad now. I don't have what is normal in my life. I can see why many people start intense projects but don't finish them. If it weren't for all the people back home who are working on this trek I don't know if I could finish. They give me the light to find my way to reach down inside myself to find that hidden reservoir that is said to be in all of us, to bring up the energy to enable me to continue despite the loneliness and depression.*

On the road I have tried to go faster, do more, get there quicker. I have not been very smart doing this, as the temperature for the last 12 days has been just around 95 degrees. So I'm really punishing my body. The loneliness is terrible. It's the same kind of loneliness of the single parent. I just want this to be over. I haven't felt this lonely since my wife died. I need to reach out to someone.

We're now into the 10th week. I am tired, exhausted, hurting. I am looking forward to getting back to life again, to thinking more clearly. My heart and passion are in the right place. God gives me the strength to continue. He has been with me all the way, carried me part of the way. What an emotional roller coaster. If not for my son Chris, J. Marie, Dr. Roth, John Pope, Greg Dittrich, Tim Forsythe, Rick Marklund, Larry Kline, Perry Williams, Mitch White, my son and daughter, Jason and Teri Sue, and others, I would not have been able to do this.

I wanted to be able to do this as a team effort. We need to set aside colors and religions, start fresh, and make a difference. I have opened a door. We can all do it if we put our minds to it. If we wait until tomorrow, and the next tomorrow, and the next tomorrow, we will postpone the good for too long. I am glad to have been able to play a small part in helping more than 35 million people have their needs discussed in the hopes that their dreams can come true, especially for the more than 22 million children in that number.

Michael asked me to say something positive. I looked at him blankly and said, "Like what?" He said not to worry, we won't include this. I looked at him. Something snapped me back to my purpose. I responded, "Yes, you will. If people are to learn that the ordinary person can do the extraordinary, they have to see it and feel it." People needed to see this dark side too. I wasn't Superman, just a man. An ordinary man. A struggling man. A single-parent caregiver man. Just like everyone else, I needed purpose and meaning in life, and my kids, all kids, this cause, gave me purpose and meaning.

After writing in my diary and climbing into bed, I offered a prayer, asking God to bless all the children and their families, asking for guidance and healing. I heard myself saying, "Let's make a difference. Let's do it today. Tomorrow is too late."

Day 69
Route: "Welcome to Georgia"
Weather: Sunny and warm.
Comment: Each step is more difficult because traffic encroaches on what little space there is on the side of the road.

DAY 69: TUESDAY, JULY 9

I started the day early and sore. I felt better as I crossed the state line. We were about three days away from Marietta where Chris and Jason were born. As I passed the WELCOME TO GEORGIA sign I knew we were going to make it. Chris informed me that we were nearly a full day ahead of schedule! I knew it would be difficult on Thursday and Friday of this week because of the traffic, which meant long days of taking it slow and easy. I predicted I would be jumping off to the side of the road many times.

Day 70
Route: Finish in Dalton, Georgia.
Weather: Warm and humid
Comment: Busy traffic on the highway. I wonder if we will make it to Atlanta.

DAY 70: WEDNESDAY, JULY 10

I spent another day dodging trucks and cars. It was a long, grueling day. It was very hot (what else?) and I got a lot of sun on my legs. My ankles felt better, especially with the ankle supports that I finally started wearing.

A group of runners passed me early in the day. We introduced ourselves. They were from England and France and were practicing for Atlanta and the Summer Olympics. I asked them if they were in the Olympics and they just said that I might see them on TV in the next week or so. I thought that perhaps the Olympics had come to us. Maybe we could have an event called the MegaMarathon in the years ahead.

Chris and I arrived in Dalton, Georgia, late in the afternoon. J. Marie Fieger of our PR firm, Nemer Fieger and Associates, called and informed us that on Sunday afternoon the media planned to meet with me near Atlanta. CNN and *60 Minutes* were showing interest also. We certainly had a heartbeat now, and it was a good thing – the finish line was literally days away.

I was sick all night. I also pulled a muscle in my upper back so I had difficulty breathing. I didn't feel well and I didn't believe it was food poisoning, as the feeling had persisted for nearly a week. Route 41 had turned into a bit nicer road but there still was no shoulder to run on.

Chris and I spent the evening watching the All Star baseball game. This was one of our family traditions and we sure did enjoy it. While we were watching television, Chris asked me if anyone knew how hard it is to do what we are doing. I said probably not. The physical? Yes. The emotional? I didn't think so.

"As Terry's cardiologist, I just knew that I couldn't stop him. He had a dream and he was going to see it through no matter what the consequences might be. He was going to make a difference in the lives of children. He was going to speak for them. Even though Terry had had a heart attack, he was going to somehow get to Atlanta, some two thousand miles away and I wasn't going to be able to stop him ... so I joined him with his dream."

—Dr. Lyle J. Swenson, M.D.

Interventional Cardiology Specialist

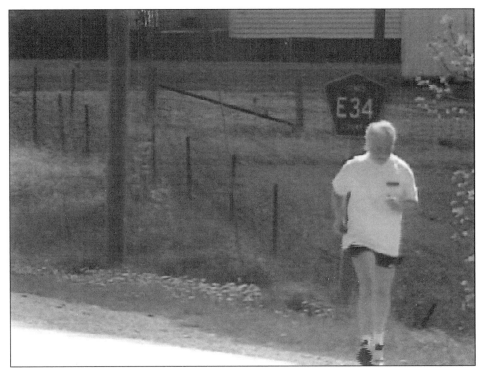

CHAPTER 17

DAYS 71 THROUGH 75

Day 71
Route: Dalton to Cartersville, Georgia.
Weather: Very hot
Comment: Hundreds of well wishers greet us on the highway. The end is close.

DAY 71: THURSDAY, JULY 11

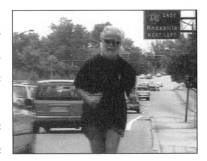

It was a difficult day. Before I left the hotel I talked with WTCH, a radio station in Atlanta. They planned to broadcast the interview today.

As usual, Chris drove ahead to see what the road was like beyond Dalton. In the meantime, I carried my water bottles and some food stuffed in my pockets as Chris drove to Dalton. When he returned, he told me I would have to be extra wary of the traffic. Highway 41, which had figured prominently in our plans, was not what we had anticipated. This particular highway goes all the way into Atlanta, and the media had already been alerted that we would be coming in by that route. So, we had to stick with Highway 41.

Chris was right. The highway from Dalton to Cartersville was terrible. The lines of traffic were long and continuous. I ducked cars and trucks constantly to hang on to my unbeaten dodge ball record. My opponents had many opportunities to beat me on that stretch, but I prevailed. I still had the last laugh. I stumbled and ran for more than thirty miles. Chris and I finished just outside of Cartersville after a full day in the sun. Michael joined us again and planned to stay until Monday to continue his filming of the MegaMarathon and to provide some much needed company.

Day 72
Route: End in Kennesaw, north of Marietta, Georgia
Weather: Hot as usual
Comment: More supporters line the highway. I really think we will make it.

DAY 72: FRIDAY, JULY 12

I made it to Kennesaw, Georgia, in one piece. Because of the heavy traffic, the going was slow, but apart from the danger of being hit by a car or truck, it was a relatively pleasant day. I spoke to WLDS radio in Alton, Illinois, again. I had spoken on the air to the Alton community previously in June. I updated WLDS, and Chris and I shared favorite stories.

We expected the next day's Run to Marietta to be slow as well, but with the finish line in sight, I was eager to keep moving. By Sunday I would run into the City of Atlanta, and then Monday travel the final miles to the official entrance at Centennial Park. I couldn't wait!

Day 73
Route: Kennesaw into Marietta, Georgia.
Weather: Hot, hot, hot
Comment: seeing old friends that I use to know when I lived in Atlanta and introducing
those friends to the friends that flew to Atlanta to be part of the Event.

DAY 73: SATURDAY, JULY 13

The miles into Marietta, a sprawling city just north of Atlanta, were tougher than usual. The weather was blistering hot and I was more tired than I thought possible. To top it off, I had an upset stomach.

Chris and I were supposed to be interviewed on the highway by the Marietta newspaper, but the ongoing Olympic news kept all the reporters too busy to meet with us. Michael joined us eager for many hours filming the finale for his documentary. Chris and I spent several of these final hours before our touchdown with him filming me running through neighborhoods and downtown Atlanta. Michael kept me busy running all over the place. Atlanta has quite a few hills and I swear he found every one of them. I think I ran as much for him on Saturday as I normally do on any given day, I covered almost double the miles if I included Michael's filming. Tomorrow will be another long day of filming as well. It was grueling but worth it, I reminded myself. The purpose of the Run was to get the word out and Michael's documentary would go a long way toward that goal.

My old friends Otis Courtney and Greg Dittrich from Minneapolis joined us for the afternoon. My son Jason also arrived with his friends, Eric and Jeremy. The visitors provided instant healing. Chris was very happy to see his brother and some friends.

I hoped some of my old friends living in Atlanta would join us Sunday night. These were friends whom I hadn't seen in more than fifteen years. With the Olympics in town, I expected some of them might be busy helping out or they might just be out of town. Hopefully, some would show up at the Holiday Inn in Marietta. For Saturday night, though, I decided to find my bed as early as possible. Sleep would be important for tomorrow's arrival. I desperately needed *some* sleep.

Day 74
Route: Depart Marietta and head into Atlanta, host of the Summer Olympics.
Weather: Hot, of course.
    Comment: I feel a wonderful sense of satisfaction and hope to have made a difference.

DAY 74: SUNDAY, JULY 14

THE FIRST FINISH LINE

My right ankle hurt when I awoke, as did my left knee. Otherwise I was OK. Chris made me breakfast and readied all the liquid I was supposed to consume for the day.

We hit the road early. The sun was bright and ready for my upcoming entrance. It was hard to believe this morning was a Sunday. Didn't this town ever sleep? The traffic seemed heavy enough for a Saturday night. I was exhilarated in a way I hadn't been since the morning of day 1. Excited, I began to flow on the fuel of adrenaline. As I continued my early morning Run my mood kept elevating and I began to feel better and better – so good, in fact, that I felt like sprinting the rest of the way. But I didn't. I wore a wonderful grin on my face instead. At last, the piece of cake had arrived. It was wonderful to feel this good again.

I traveled the narrow and heavily trafficked Highway 41. As the day grew hotter and more humid it also seemed to grow longer. That didn't surprise me. We had had that kind of weather since the first of June and it sapped my strength more and more with each additional stride. I was as accustomed to it as a person can get, I believe.

As I ran, I played the game of jumping on the highway for one hundred feet and then jumping off for the same distance while traffic went by. I forced myself to keep my eyes on the oncoming traffic at all times. One slip, not paying attention for one moment and I would be a goner. Seemed like I had played this game all the way down from the Twin Cities, and I didn't want to lose in the last few seconds of regulation time.

The sun grew even hotter. I had had more than enough sun for an entire summer. I tried to protect myself but after awhile it became very difficult. Wearing a hat was usually impossible because of the passing big trucks, which produced such drafts that no hat would stay on. I ended up with a bare head, no matter how I started out. Sunscreen was great except on my face – after running a short while, sweat carried it into my eyes where it burned fiercely and blurred my vision. I finally decided I would rather go without sun protection and see the traffic than be lathered in sunscreen and possibly dead. We approached Atlanta in the middle of the afternoon. The climbing humidity and the sun were draining my strength. I wanted to run into the city with arms held high and a big smile, but the smile was all I could do. I felt really tired and my ankles were killing me again.

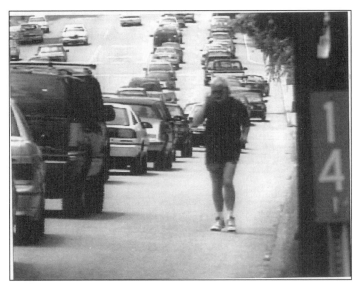

As we were getting close to the finish line, Chris parked the car to run the last few miles with me. About a mile from the capitol, with a sudden, anxious jolt, I was struck with a fear that we might be going the wrong way.

Then we passed the double fence around the Olympic Village and the obviously heavy security; we were going the right direction after all. It seemed so strange to be running with the Atlanta skyline behind me, after so many miles on country and rural roads where the only tall objects were trees and mountains.

Finally, we rounded our last street corner and there, straight ahead, were the steps up to the capitol entrance – the Finish Line.

We reached the Finish Line to the cheers of a crowd that included many familiar faces. My daughter Teri Sue, my son Jason, J. Marie, Zak, Greg, Otis, Eric and Jeremy, and Andy. They had all flown in to witness the end of the Run. Even faces I had not met cheered us on the last few steps. Lights were flashing. Bulbs were popping. Strobes were glaring. Photographers and television cameras were there to record our finish.

Finishing the Run felt great, but also anticlimactic. More than two thousand miles of well-traveled road were behind us. We had made it. I had made it. Who would have thought it? The sun was blazingly hot and the air dripped with humidity, but I didn't mind anymore. I had made it to Atlanta. But this was only the first of two finishes. The media wanted another time with me, the next day, at Centennial Park.

We stayed (where else?) at the Marietta Holiday Inn the entire time we were in Atlanta. The hotel also gave us complimentary rooms for any other guests who might fly in to join us through the weekend. They sure were lifesavers.

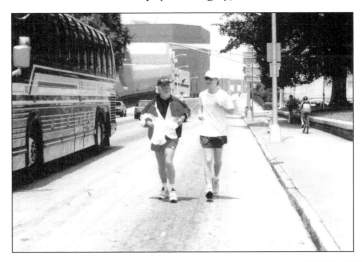

Day 75
Route: Retrace some steps, run course through Atlanta to the finish line.
Weather: Hot, but who cares.
   Comment: We thought this was the end of our journey, but it was only the beginning.

DAY 75: MONDAY, JULY 15

THE SECOND FINISH LINE

We finished a second time on Monday, which I realized ironically brought us back on schedule. I asked Chris to join me. It was another beautiful day. Chris and I retraced our steps of the previous day. Piece of cake.

As we ran back into Atlanta the streets seemed less busy – quiet even. It felt eerie, as though the whole city was waiting for us somewhere. There was a smooth glide to our running. Nothing really ached anymore. This was really the Final Run. This was it. This was now fun. The corner where we turned left was just ahead, and our surroundings still seemed strangely quiet. Another corner, then, the last.

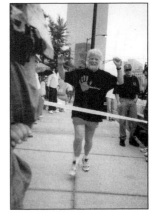

As we made the turn I could see the Finish Line – a real one – stretched across the road ahead of us. Wow! Everyone was waiting. I couldn't believe the crowd. It was huge. As we came to the Finish Line Chris let me cross first and break the tape.

Television cameras were everywhere. Hugs were now plentiful after more than ten weeks and more than two thousand miles. I went from one interview to the next. It felt great to get the message out. Organizations like Save The Children Coalition and Children First were represented, along with many others.

Some of my old friends from the days when we lived in Marietta joined us in the celebration. We had a great time and it really helped Chris and me to begin to celebrate our own landing. We were done. We had really finished. *Or was this just the beginning?*

The 1996 Olympic Games were set to start in a couple of days. Many people said they wished I could stay for the Games, maybe participate in the Opening Ceremonies. I just looked at them and wondered, *didn't they realize I have been running for seventy-five consecutive days?* The only things I could think about at that moment were hot baths and warm beds. I would be perfectly content watching the Games on TV, assuming I didn't sleep the next week straight through. Besides, in the back of my mind I asked: *are people cheering for the purpose or the physical feat?* The Olympics would be wonderful to watch tomorrow. But that day, July 15, belonged to Run '96. We were honored that the Mayor of Atlanta and other dignitaries met us and congratulated us for our Olympic-sized effort.

The media also gathered at the entrance to Centennial Park, and what a wondrous national and international mix it was. WXIA-TV, WAGA-TV, WGNA, WXIA and the Japanese, Finnish, and Mexican networks, all with reporters. The Twin Cities were represented too. The

Star Tribune came to interview me, as did Minneapolis' KARE 11 Television. They all give us a marvelous Olympic-size Atlanta welcome.

Finished. The two thousand mile Run on behalf of children and single-parent families was over. But my hope was that this was just the beginning of what we can do for our children.

Later, we were honored with a party at Planet Hollywood. Our large Twin City contingent sat in a special guest section. Bright lights were on us as Chris and I were presented with a wonderful proclamation and a Certificate of Honor from Mayor Campbell. This, too, was televised. The cameras focused in and out and stayed with us until we left Atlanta later on.

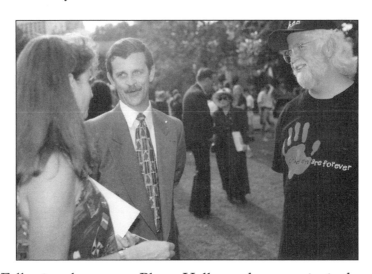

Following the party at Planet Hollywood we were invited to a special function at Piedmont Park hosted by Polar Heart Monitors and Mayor Campbell. The occasion was the ceremonial unveiling of a new statue, *The Last Meter*, sculpted by Eno and dedicated to Atlanta for the Olympics. Among the many dignitaries at the event were Ms. Cara H. Axam, president and chief executive officer of CODA, Mr. Tony Harmon, president of Polar Electro Inc., Mr. Kosti Rasinpera, the Honorable General Secretary of the Finnish Olympic Committee, Ms. Sandra Perfmutter, executive director of the President's Council on Physical Fitness and Sports, and Mr. G. Joseph Prendergast, co-chairman of CODA.

It was a great Olympic theme and a wonderful celebration. In my own private thoughts I felt I truly knew what the last meter means. I questioned myself during this Run, just as parents question themselves on how they are doing, wondering if they are doing what is right and best for their kids, and, most agonizingly, whether they all will make it.

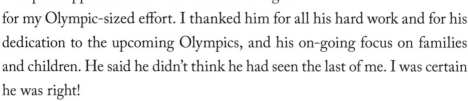

It was wonderful to see the proud, beaming faces of my kids. I couldn't picture a better reward than to see the pride radiating from them. That alone was an incredible thrill.

Soon after the function was over, Mayor Campbell approached me and thanked me again for my Olympic-sized effort. I thanked him for all his hard work and for his dedication to the upcoming Olympics, and his on-going focus on families and children. He said he didn't think he had seen the last of me. I was certain he was right!

Following the Piedmont Park unveiling ceremony we were off to a private dinner hosted by Polar Heart Monitors. What an incredibly event-packed day! Adrenaline must have kept me going through it all.

We had already packed our things and all that was left to do was get to the Atlanta airport. During the Run I had lost my checkbook and my wallet and identification so my friends vouched for me. Thank goodness security was not as tight then as it later became. I just wanted to get home. We boarded the plane and flew north to Minneapolis via Sun Country Airlines' last flight. What a day. *Sleep*, I kept thinking. *I can't wait.*

It had been a great ten weeks and I was still on my high, but I was ready to come down to earth. I was feeling the long Run and just wanted to sleep, to sleep soundly perhaps for the first time in many weeks. But there was to be none of that yet. On the flight I gave a little girl my Polar hat and her mom cried. It turned out that she was a single parent and she was greatly appreciative of our efforts.

As we flew back home I leaned back. I finally got to close my eyes. But I couldn't sleep. My mind surveyed the panoramic sweep of the past seventy-five days. As I thought back I asked myself, *how did I do it? Can it be true that I have just run over two thousand miles in seventy-five consecutive days?* And yet, I wasn't exerting the effort alone. I ran as a member of several communities: the support community in the Twin Cities that made it possible, the community of towns along the way, and, most importantly, the community of single parents and their children, for whom I ran and who cheered me along the route.

I had begun with a vision that became a mission to eradicate a problem plaguing every American community and school, affecting more than half of our children. How do we do it? It is first a local problem, a grassroots problem that must first be tackled there. Often we feel poorly equipped to solve the problem at this level, thinking there must be a national solution. But we are a nation of communities, and what our local communities do to address the problem will shape the policy of our nation. There is too much wrangling about the topic and too much competition for tax dollars to rely on any kind of top-down government action. That leaves the private (for-profit) sector and the philanthropic (not-for-profit) and the pre-school and K-12 sectors. But mostly it leaves the families themselves. It means that individuals are going to have to step up to the plate and take their turns at bat in terms of responsibly working with their communities, their families, their spouses, their kids, and themselves.

It was late in the Twin Cities as we landed. It was wonderful to be back after almost three months on the highway, no matter what the hour. We were all exhausted. But then, as I left the plane and entered the terminal I quickly realized that the night was not yet over. Hundreds of friends were waiting for us. Lights flashed and cameras rolled. Signs and banners were everywhere. The adrenaline began pumping again. The hugs I had longed for over these last ten weeks came all at once. The *Children Are Forever* choir was there and they sang two beautiful songs, one they had written themselves. What a delightful welcome!

They sang:

We are the adults of tomorrow,
You're our example of today,
You'd better watch what you say
And be careful what you do
'Cause we've got big eyes
And we are looking at you
Just for today be good examples,
Which means, of course,
You have to mend your ways.
For your positives should
Outweigh your negatives,
And we're tired of hearing
All those naughty adjectives.
So we're here with a plea
As you can plainly see.
So watch what you do!
We're looking at you.

I was presented with flowers, a bottle of champagne, and plenty of balloons. People asked me to speak. What could I say?

"Thank you, thank you, and thank you. It is wonderful to be back among so many friends. You all made it worthwhile. Thinking of you every day

helped me to keep going. You made it all worthwhile. Thank you from the bottom of my heart. I can't thank you enough for your support, your efforts, and your prayers. Because of your work you have enabled lives along the Run to change in positive ways. Because of your work we will continue to bring positive change to the problems associated with single parent families. This is not the end; it is the beginning. Thank you, and God Bless you."

After many more exhausted thank-yous and hugs, I went off to my warm bed with happy thoughts.

The long-term effects of two thousand miles of the Run, justified every moment, every step, and every ache. We affected the lives of many, many people. I knew kids everywhere would be helped. Single parents had been given new hope. God carried me many times. All the team members helped in so many ways. My children were proud of me and I was proud of them. My son Chris was superb. Teri Sue, Jason, Andy, Mike, Kim, and Charlie all helped immeasurably. Charlie enthusiastically came to me as if I had just had a long day at work. I returned home thinking there were so many volunteers to thank and so much more work to do. My trek was about single parents and their kids and even more, it was about all our everyday heroes.

But first, I slept.

EPILOGUE

When I crossed the finish line in Atlanta in July 1996, I thought I had done my part to give back and my work was finished. Hadn't I made my point about the importance of helping single parents? I thought I had recognized, rallied and recruited "everyday heroes" to help the kids of single parents realize their dreams. If newspaper ink, magazine pages, and TV and radio time are the measure, then I had more than my fair share of fifteen minutes of fame.

In fact, after the Run, I was feeling so hopeful I tried to set up a Return Run from Atlanta to Minneapolis for the end of the summer. Evidently, my physical fatigue had sapped my ability to think rationally!

After the Run, of course, I was soon yesterday's news. I doggedly tried to sustain the positive energy and focus of the Run, to channel it into meaningful projects in which everyone could participate. My friend Peter Jessen volunteered to help. He, too, is a single parent, and we share many of the same values. He had wonderful ideas about how we could move forward. Projects were lined up. We had some tentative commitments. But it was too soon for me.

I "crashed and burned" emotionally. The Run's physical and emotional toll was too much for me. It was little consolation to know that what I was going through was common among many world-class athletes, deep sea-divers, and others with "mountain-top" experiences. They rarely talk about the emotional tailspin that follows intense and prolonged physical exertion and now I understand why. I entered the hospital near the end of the summer and spent seven weeks there, healing my body and recovering from a nasty bout of depression.

Looking back, I can see I was a bit naïve to think my Run by itself would have a lasting impact. I have since learned that events like mine get things started, but are not sustaining. My Run was interesting, even inspiring, for a short time, but we are all tethered to a fickle media monster that needs to be fed something fresh twenty-four hours a day, seven days a week. Yes, I had a worthy cause, and yes, I had found a photogenic – perhaps crazy – way to grab some attention for everyday heroes. But back then, I didn't have a good answer to "what's next?" I wasn't even sure that I would actually finish the Run, and so I certainly couldn't predict that I would have a lasting impact. Instead, I ran on faith, and here's what I know about faith: Faith sees the invisible, believes the incredible, and receives the impossible. While I was in the hospital, I had time to listen, and God said He had a few more marathons for me.

The Run was just a warm up, I think – it may not have changed the world forever, but it certainly ignited new passions in me to create sustainable resources that help parents help their kids live up to their full potential. This time, I am building a team with more legs than just mine in the form of the *Heroes & Dreams Foundation*, a National Heritage Foundation

My vision now is to forever link the commercial success of businesses to the social success of their customers and employees. This is a popular notion, sometimes called socially-responsible business or social entrepreneurship. Through the *Heroes & Dreams Foundation*, we promote two programs that simultaneously meet the hard-nosed, measurable marketing objectives of retail and manufacturing brand managers while simultaneously directing more money and resources to schools and other nonprofits.

Our first program is Labels for Learning TM, which is an automated label redemption program designed to bring schools more money. The second is the HeroCard TM, which rewards volunteers for their time through discounts at national retailers. We call these programs cause-media channels, and we think programs like ours create new, sustainable partnerships between business, government, and nonprofit sectors. One of our unique contributions is our accommodation of each partner's core mission: No one is asked to do anything they are not already committed to, and this makes the partnership natural and authentic, not contrived or dependent.

Epilogue

While our cause-media programs at the *Heroes & Dreams Foundation* help all nonprofits, you won't be surprised to know that my personal passion is helping to fix our education system. One third of our kids are not prepared to learn when they start kindergarten and – no surprise – the same proportion fails to graduate. Our kids' plight is worse in urban areas, with fifty percent failing to graduate. Bill Milliken, a thirty-year veteran of the marathon to help at-risk kids through schools, says America has faced a "dropout epidemic" for decades in his wonderful book, The Last Dropout: Stop the Epidemic! Despite piles of research that shows that education, among other things, creates more productive citizens and less crime, we remain unable – which really means *unwilling* – to get education right.

I am too old and stubborn to just tip toe around the margins of change. Because I am a business guy, I appreciate the power of the free market and its inherent ability to achieve "Big Idea" goals with efficiency and effectiveness. The business organization is – potentially – an ideal partner for social change. We simply need to remove the social and mental barriers we erected so long ago and open our eyes to new possibilities that recognize the importance of education to our kids, our companies' competitiveness, and our nation's future – and how it is all intimately intertwined.

My Run began with a passion to help kids and their parents. I endured a heavy physical and mental toll on that odyssey, and at the end of the Run I truly did not know whether I had made the lives of American kids and struggling parents any better. But I do know that I am a better person for having tried. If I have learned anything during my life, it is that I cannot change the world, but I can change *MY* world. You don't have to run seventy-five marathons in seventy-five consecutive days to make a difference in the lives of kids; instead, it's the little things that are often the most heroic.

REFLECTIONS - LOOKING BACK

American businesses today are abuzz with their latest "Big bets." Corporations talk about big bets; strategic leaders make big bets with their divisions and expect individual employees to commit to big bets for the next fiscal year. These "big bets" are usually challenges with the potential to cause damage through failure. While great reward awaits success, that success is far from guaranteed. There is always risk. And sometimes that risk is a missed opportunity or a regression - if the company doesn't take on this big bet, they might lose market share, or see a drop in customer satisfaction and loyalty. The big bet affects the bottom line through failure or success. But the most important aspect of the big bet is the lack of neutrality. Doing nothing is not an option.

Are we, as a community, faced with big bets? If so, do we see them and are we acting upon them?

I saw the world on the long two thousand miles to Atlanta. I felt the heart beat of people who shared their personal feelings, their pain, their frustration and their soul. It was such a powerful experience. They knew that I was real and that I was struggling to accomplish my Run for them. These parents saw in me their own daily marathons and saw my struggles and success as their own.

The big bets outside the corporate world, our children, followed me on my trek each day. As I challenged the viewing audience on live TV one day, I asked the question about our future as a country and as a society. I posed the question that if our children are the future of our country then *why don't we have a Secretary of Children?* We have a Secretary of Labor, Energy, and Defense, but not a federal or state cabinet position on what is our most important asset. It makes all the sense in the world. If our children are our future, then why don't we have a strong representation of such a valuable asset? We don't. Our kids know it. They told me over and over again. They feel alone. Our kids are looking for someone to run down their highways for them and with them. Parents are absent. Parents are arguing and not communicating to their children. Fathers, more than mothers, are absent. Single parents are the majority, not the minority. We are failing our children. We are failing ourselves.

What this country needs to do is *refocus* our priorities. Do what is right. Our political system needs substantial repair. Our representatives in Washington are political. It's not that they don't want to do what is right – most do. However, the politicians roll with the punches, follow the crowd, and worry about their own skin and not the good of the people.

We need strong leaders, working together, to get what needs to be done, done. Our children need to be at the forefront. We need to start with early childhood education. It has been said that early childhood education should start right after a child is potty trained. Why not even earlier? That training must be done by whoever is available for our children, whether it is a parent, a grandparent, or even a neighbor. If we don't take up the task of educating our children, then we all lose. And to educate our children, we need to ensure they are not distracted by health problems, whether illness or hunger. Again, we slip badly on this front. It is obvious that education, the entire realm of education, needs to be transformed. We are behind the times in how we present education. Our children are getting short changed. Along with this critical point are a majority of parents today who are "single parents." Single parents, all parents, need the services of daycare or what I call assisted daycare, as many, many parents today cannot afford such a luxury for taking care of their children.

In *American Business: The Last Hurrah?* I wrote that the role of education in today's society is the cornerstone for the future – a chance to positively change the world. Our country and our people can prosper and grow if education is paramount in their lives and the educational process for each individual continues with their each and every heartbeat. A present dilemma facing our society – thirty-seven percent of our fourth graders cannot read (one half of minorities), one in four students will not graduate from high school, and U.S. eighth-graders are underachievers in science and math, ranking 17th and 18th respectively, when compared to eighth-graders in other developed nations.

Education needs reform. Access to college is not a major problem. Success is. The four-year graduation rate for a baccalaureate degree is a meager thirty-four percent and the six-year graduation rate isn't all that much better at fifty-six percent. The retention rate for low-income and minority students at many universities is much lower than for their peers. These low-income and minority students get through the door but leave before completing their education. Remedial and developmental course attendance continues to climb.

Sharing my thoughts with the thoughts of others, a fundamentally new way of thinking in American schools is needed. The model in place today is a remnant of the nineteenth Century. It might have worked for a long time, and that is debatable, but it is doubtful that it will measure up to the challenges of the twenty-first century. This country faces challenges in the organization, governance, financing, and accountability of education.

Reforms like the federal No Child Left Behind law should make it easier to marry elementary and secondary education to higher education by setting standards for what high-school students need to know to prepare for college. But while some states are seeking to promote K-16 cooperation, too often they don't go far enough. The powerful teacher union resists, saying it can't be done without more money and resources rather than stopping to figure out how to do it with existing funding and resources. Never have so many schools had so much and achieved so much less. In far too many places, high school is either a place to bide one's time until college or an extension of middle school rather than a preparation for adulthood. Advanced students get bored and tune out intellectually. Others are never challenged to acquire the skills and education needed beyond life in high school.

The new educational approach will require the entrepreneurial drive and the venture capital of the private sector. It also requires the energy and ideas of the private sector that depends so much on educated citizens. What is needed, indeed, is educational and private sector entrepreneurship. It is unreasonable to expect government, at any level, to introduce fundamental change in such a fundamental enterprise, as that is not the job of government. It takes fresh ideas and fresh faces – qualities government seldom possesses when so far removed from the local communities where education takes place. It requires a willingness to take risks, to which government is averse, and that also is not the government's job. It requires true leadership from those in schools who help fashion the next generation of American education and the allowance of local parents, business and citizens to have a say on developing accountability measures for the schools to which they send their children.

Yes, the big bet I see is to build a strong foundation for our children to survive, flourish, and to be successful in their individual lives. We are continuing to tear apart this existing foundation with inadequate programs and political indecisions. The consequences spell catastrophe. A strong, trusting public-private partnership can avert such catastrophe. It begins with parents, first and foremost, being involved in their children's lives – including at school, church and in the community. If we do this, the community of parents will create a world of possibilities for their children.

Wouldn't it be nice if we <u>all</u> could dream together and believe together.

ACKNOWLEDGEMENTS

I could not have made this Run or written this book alone. It was a team effort. I could not have done it without the incredible support I received before, during and after the Run. I don't want to be glib and say thanks to all of you, you know who you are, and let it go at that. You're too important to me, and this is my book – I'm going to say "thank you" in print no matter what, so get over it!

I get to start with my special thanks to my three kids, Teri Sue, Chris and Jason. Kids: So much has started with you and because of you. You three have been the bedrock of my life since your mom died, and you have kept me going when I didn't think I could. You each know that without you the MegaMarathon (thank you, Denny Green, for naming it) could not have taken place. Without your love and support, and those times we laughed until our faces hurt, my crazy training and work schedules would have done us in. May you, my children, the lights of my life, continue to grow and develop and pace yourselves for the marathons of daily life – may you always run them as well as you do today. You remain an inspiration to me, your proud father and good friend, as well as to the many others whose lives you have affected so positively.

Next, a few leaders of leaders deserve special attention. J. Marie Fieger, of the public relations firm Nemer Fieger & Associates, is the Run's MVP, our guardian angel, the driving force behind our publicity success and the glue that held the support crew together in the Twin Cities. Scott Meier, the "connector" (thank you, Oprah) between my body and the Run, who worked with me throughout seventeen months of early mornings, self-doubt and fickle weather to prepare my body. And Drs. Meghabhuti Roth, David Thorson and Lyle Swenson, who designed the physical regimen I followed that kept me alive. Dr. Roth also provided additional training for my mental and emotional management, and he helped me handle the overall stress of the Run. Dr. Roth taught me how to deal with the dreaded "walls," both the traditional one (more myth than reality) and the special one encountered during long physical exertions (very real indeed). Greg Dittrich and his father, Duane, put together the vehicles to move the team each day on the road. Greg, Gene Larkin and Perry Williams gave me critical spiritual strength at times of distress. Tim Forsythe and his company, Forsythe Appraisal, were there for me every single time I needed encouragement. I am particularly grateful to Rick Marklund for giving me the opportunity to continue my vision for kids. The work he accomplished with Hyperport and the vision he had for improving the lives of all people through the various Hyperport projects have a positive impact on the lives of millions of people worldwide. Finally, I am grateful to my friend and co-author Peter Jessen, with whom I have worked with on various management consulting assignments. He joined me for ten days, took notes as he listened to me talk about the Run and reviewed some of the fifty-plus videotapes taken during the Run. He faithfully captured the spirit of what it was like to be me on the Run, and he helped me organize my diary notes into something readable. I've said it for many years, Peter, and I'll say for many more – you're the best. And as for Jeff Turner and Kyle Gearhart who took all of our writings and massaged it into a meaningful story, I thank you both. And to Tim VandeSteeg, a magical independent director and producer in the Hollywood film community who believed in my story and will put the story in a documentary tentatively called "My Run" to be followed by a feature film titled "Pushing Life", I thank you. And finally, I promise, to my business partner who prodded me many times when I wanted to let my story get stale and place it back on the shelf. So much to thank Brad Thompson for.

Whew – fast forward the video to a gray and windy morning on the side of an empty country road. The Run has begun and times are hard. You have to meet my road crew, a group of the greatest kids I have ever had the pleasure to know. My road crew consisted of Kim Doverspike, Andy Stemig, Mike Kearney and my sons Chris and Jason Hitchcock. The home crew members were J. Marie Fieger, Perry Williams, Greg Dittrich, Otis Courtney, and Teri Sue Hitchcock.

Special thanks to my son Chris, who single-handedly shouldered the road work to keep me going during weeks five through eleven. He was a one-man MASH unit extraordinaire when we had to reorganize midway through the Run. He stayed the course, fed me, clothed me and found places to rest and sleep. Chris never let me forget that even though I was just an ordinary man, and thus had to follow the doctors' orders to survive, I was also extraordinary. I was Dad, a guy, he said, who showed him the meaning and grace of a larger purpose, the joy of trying, the thrill of being in the arena and the transcendent power of love. That was a special time, son, when the hard times brought out the best in us.

Thank you also to each and every child who sang in the Children Are Forever Choir. Remembering the sound of your voices was an inspiration to me when I really needed it. You were there for my send-off and for my homecoming. During fundraisers your songs inspired others to help sustain our effort financially so I could keep running. Many thanks to Roberta Davis, the choir director, and Bev Asher, who helped write lyrics. "The Children Are Watching" themes figure prominently in our current work at the *Heroes & Dreams Foundation*.

Corporate America didn't stand on the sidelines, either. During my training, I used primarily Nike shoes, although Nike was not a sponsor, and during the Run I used specially made New Balance shoes. I also used BowFlex equipment during the training as I needed to continually work on building my stamina, endurance and strength.

The sponsors who provided equipment did so out of a belief in the goals of the Run. Given the different levels of giving to the Run, we divided our sponsors into three groups: Gold, Silver and Bronze.

Gold Sponsors:

> Breathe Right
> Domino's Pizza, Inc.
> Minnesota Twins Baseball
> Petters Warehouse Direct
> Polar Heart Rate Monitors
> Rollerblade, Inc.
> RUDS, Inc.
> Strategic Alliances, Inc.
> Tires Plus
> New Balance
> Wigwam Socks

Silver Sponsors:

> Head Lites
> Knott's Camp Snoopy
> Mini Pac
> SSMG & Provident Worldwide
> Subway Sandwich & Salad Shops
> XLR8 & UltraGel

Bronze Sponsors:

> AT&T Wireless Services
> Banana Boat Products
> Bennett's Cycle
> Dial
> Gargoyles Performance Eyewear
> Homepage
> Natural Ovens
> Natus Products

Acknowledgements

Northwest Health Clubs (now LifeTime Fitness)

PR Nutrition

Perkins Family Restaurant & Bakery

Spirit Water Co.

Super America

WFTC (Fox) Twin Cities

West Link Paging

Post-Run Platinum Special Good Samaritan Award:

Holiday Inns of America

Others who helped and contributed:

Sky Harbour Inns

Francie's Bed and Breakfast, DuQuoin, Ill

Let me just take a moment to share some of my personal heroes with you. I call them heroes because they have, in many ways, impacted my life. Now I want to honor them, sort of a personal roast if you will.

- Minnie and Harvey Bolton. Grandparents. My grounding. My home. My enchanted village.
- Buddy and Estelle McWilliams. Uncle and Aunt. Parents of four sons: David, Alexander Jr., Kevin and Gary. A guiding light of parenting.
- Genevieve Beatrice Bolton. Mother. Multi-talented. Unlimited musical array. Loving. Gave me up in order to provide for me.
- Mollie and Frank Fecteau. Mary Ann and Tim's mom and dad. Wonderful example of love, affection and natural honesty. Parenting supreme.
- Joseph Brennan. My coach, friend and scout leader. He was my anchor through the "growing up" years and helped me to believe in myself.

- John Pope. A constant friend. A valued confessor and an impartial judge. A stern rudder, always there for me. A spouse and soul mate for Marlene.

- Richard Yutendale. Long time friend. Loyal. Dick and Marie transcend time.

- Rich and Judy Adamkiewicz. From counselor to Daytona to dedicated teachers to restless travelers. Always there.

- David and Jean Kronemeyer. Extraordinaire in all aspects. They receive straight "As" for their passion for life, helping others, and faith in mankind.

- "Charlie" the dog. Helped me train for the long days on the road and the sleepless nights of pain and questioning. He was "man's best friend". He was my friend.

- Vi Turner. She is everyone's "Granny". Adored by so many. We all miss Papa, Vi's partner and husband for many years.

- Aleane White. Sue's mother. A wonderful parent and grandmother. She gave me a precious gift. Thank you.

- Richard Marklund. International Businessman. A born senator. Orator. Valued friend. World's pastor. Loving saint. Nina's best friend and husband.

- Teri Sue Hitchcock. Daughter. Confidant. Musical. Dramatist. Playwright. Teacher. Survivor. Jason's best friend and wife.

- Jason Hitchcock. Son. Expressful. Multi-talented. Explorer. Artist. Guitarist. Thinker. Playful. Colorful loving friend. Selena's best friend.

- Christian Hitchcock. Son. Heartfelt. Caring. Future poet. Athletic. Authentic. Focused. Passionate. Friend.

- Maurice Titus. Teacher. Valued friend, uncle and guide. Provider of life's daily truths.

Acknowledgements

- Brad Thompson. Loving husband of Ellen and proud parent of twins, David and Katie. Prolific writer. Wonderful mind. Friend and trusting business partner. The highest of values. An educational genius.
- Otis Courtney. A seeker of truth and purveyor of His word. An angelic voice, which he and wife Stephanie share with others.
- Greg Dittrich, his son Andrew, and his dad, Duane Dittrich. Greg leads the field in friendship, parenting and giving to others. Greg's mother and father, Pauline and Duane, raised their son to be his best.
- J. Marie Fieger and her daughter, Emelia. The queen of public relation events. The mother of supporting one's cause and the sister of providing passion to one's heart. To all, she is the best. To the rest, well, there is no one left.
- Red Skelton. Red closed each performance with "God Bless". He certainly was. We certainly are.
- Alfred Hitchcock. To me, he was "my uncle". Of course, he really was. He explored. I explored. He invested. I invested. He walked in his dreams. I ran in mine.
- Ernest Griffes. Long time confidant. Supporter of the aged and the genuine article of friendship outstanding. A leader in a long list of achievements for mankind. Carol's best friend.
- Karen and Darryl Bramer. Outstanding parents and friends/supporters of and for many. Always there. Always ready. Always.
- Stanton Hitchcock. Grandfather I did not know well but his musical and twinkling eyes and gentle touch told me, even at a young age, that I too would be blessed.
- Peter Jessen's sons – Eric, Craig and Kyle – were raised by their father, alone. That should say it all. A loving and giving father provided each son with his many talents and gifts. The world awaits.
- Dr. Robert Gillio's daughters Anna, Amy, Sophia and Maria are blessed to have shared Rob and Beth's gift of outstanding parenting.

Love abounds. Talents are nourished and grown and the world awaits Rob's next gifts from such a multi-talented mind.

- Molly Mehl. My stepdaughter. Energetic. Fun loving and high quality of caring and sharing. Couldn't ask for more. Blessed to have Molly and Ron in my life.

- Tom Peck. My stepson. Blessed to have Tom and Stacy in my life. Their sons, Ryan and Connor, are also in our lives. Mary Ann and my first grandchildren.

- Larry Kline and his two daughters, Abigail Rose and Meredith Jean. Larry wins the highest award of "parent". A heart almost too big. He would feed the world if he could. This is God's star pupil.

- Durward "Woody" Starr. A vet to the world's animals. A charitable provider. A Red Sox supporter. The best right fielder and fast break artist. A fantasy baseball invitee. Lorraine's best friend.

- David Hamelin. Hard worker and provider. Gentle giant. Will never leave a fallen comrade. Valued friend. Husband of Lucille.

- Roland "Junior" Denton. Junior could excel in any sport and succeed. Admired by entire community. An inspiration. A Yankee supporter. Pit's best friend.

- Bob Hegland. Man's best friend. Ask anyone. Solid. Charitable. A gracious friend and father to Bob, Kimberly, Dani and Dustin. Grandfather to Madison. Racquetball player supreme.

- Pastor Kent Grosser. A gentle man who delivers a powerful message. Kent is a teacher and a leader of His flock.

- Tim Forsythe. He gave. He asked not for a return but asked to make a difference. Tim was behind the long trek and created the opportunity to make the changes for our kids, parents and communities. He delivered from his heart. Tim and Mary are parents superb.

- Eric Paczosa and Jeremy Schauer. Real friends and providers of real caring. Always, always there.

Acknowledgements

- Norm Coleman. Senator of Minnesota and former Mayor of Saint Paul. A true leader. A real communicator. A real person. Real people are the foundation of our history and our future.
- Richard Barbacane. A true visionary who expects the best from our educational system and who is always ready to help us get there. He upholds all principles for education and family. He represents the kind of leadership we need for our educational system if it is to realize its full potential.
- Donna Smith. Supreme provider of family entertainment. A courageous adventurer within the film industry and a superb presenter of "stories" that have a need to be shared. The world of fantasy, adventure and comedy owes a debt of gratitude to this hero.
- Richard Salliterman. Excellent attorney. Highest of integrity. Carries the banner of fairness and honesty. A great family leader.
- Gene Larkin. Some know him for his baseball expertise and hero status. I know Gene for his enthusiasm for life, his giving to others, and his dedication to make a difference in our world. He was a World Series hero. He was and always will be a world class act.
- Zak Manuszak. A special parent. A strategic business thinker. A loyal family provider.
- Bob Blank. Theoritical and questioning mind. Great family person and trusting and solid parent. Good friend. Soul mate for Ann.
- Forler Massnick. An author. An entrepreneur. Smart. Sophisticated. Honest. Loving husband of Carrie.
- James Bowers. "Dr. Jim". Life-long friend. War hero. Pilot. Lugar collector. Guitarist.
- Harold Haynes. An important part of my earlier life. Teacher. Parent. Church leader. Community father.

- Perry Williams. Sports television announcer. Important aspect of the Run. Disciplined. Planner. To be counted on. Loyal. Best friend and spouse of Ann Pachciarek.
- Melvin Monteith. My hero. Big heart. Shortened life. Sad ending.
- Cheryl Alexander. Search business extraordinaire. Outstanding parent. World traveler. Kind and considerate. Best friend to John.
- Lil Farrar. Well thought of. A constant smile. Grandmother. Joyous. Good person.
- Leonard Przybylski. Honest. Willing to share. Supportive. Creative. Wanting to help. Admired.
- Bob Bardwell. Everyone's hero. Outstanding heart. Biggest provider to the dreams for others. God's substitute teacher.
- Al and Tina Hitchcock. Parents of Melanie and Andrew. Long lost family and missed brother for fifty years. Represents an important ingredient for the world to keep faith and focus. An admired and invaluable portion of life's future. An outstanding brother. Thanks for the new family coming into my life.
- Allan Grosh and Lynne Lancaster. Always there. Allan – racquetball champion. Father elite. Lynne – author extraordinaire. People's champion. True friends. The best of the best.
- Ron Mehl. Husband of Molly. Champion of fish and game. Will do anything for someone and will always be there for them. Thanks for the caring.
- Stacy Peck. Wife of Tom and mother of Ryan and Connor. Strong supporter of parental traditions and caring person to all those around her.
- Jim and Polly Ekern. Always there. Never without "Anything else I can do." "Do you need some help?" They represent the best example of friendship.

Acknowledgements

- Iris Waade. Talented. Creative artist. Close friend always and best friend to Sue. Loving parent for Robbie and dedicated to those in need.
- Clay Hitchcock. Missed greatly. Uncle. Surrogate best friend. Provided guidance and support for life's many issues and challenges.
- John and Dorothy Moore. Long lost and now found relatives. Canadian bound. Caring and supportive. Strong foundation for family and spiritual ties. Good friends. Good people. Sadly, a recent loss of Dorothy.
- Jim Sullivan. Great teacher and mentor. Business savvy. High principles. Strong leader. The best!
- Jesse Overton. Each day, each audience, he molds new thinking into each person's heart. A man of distinction. A person of integrity and respect. A true friend.
- David Mooney. A talented Tiger Woods shadow. Strong parenting skills. Great friend. Always there. The Smart Card industry's ambassador to the world.
- Elizabeth "Beth" Terrell. Her family's angel of mercy. Dedicated with pure honesty. A heart of golden rain drops.
- Norm Lanpher. Very simply, a great friend who has never been forgotten. A gift for life. Loving husband to Joyce.
- High School Class of 1957. Fond memories. Norm, Suzanne, David, Roddy, Shirley and Joan. Thanks.
- Greg Hewitt. A provider. Comic relief. Dreamer. Actor. Big heart.
- Jackie Robinson. A childhood hero. He had a dream. He knew he could. He never gave up. He overcame tremendous odds to live his dream.
- William G. Cash. A substitute father. Good listener. Excellent teacher.

- John Bryant. Friend. Business strategist. Spouse to Lynn and father to MacKenzie, Lauren and Kelsi.
- Ellerd Tomte. Strong business ethics. Valuable supporter. Disciplined. Good person to share life's issues with.
- John Lipps. Creative golfer. Long time friend. Father. Super new business idea creator. Good heart. Gentle giant among dreamers.
- Joseph Francis Campbell. God's teacher and loving substitute parent. Life should be guided by Joe's heart and love for others.
- Ed Sewell. Supporter for good. A counselor's counselor. True example to follow. A loving soul.
- Bob Hoffman. The legal profession's best friend. Successful leader of business and foundations. Extraordinary parent. A guide for the human soul.
- Wes Hayne. Long-term friend. Sax player extraordinary. Stock and financial expert. True business magnet. Husband of Linda and father of Tim, Jon, Chris and Mark.
- Jim Pavelle. Superb artist. Fraternity little big brother. Long lost friend.
- Fidler girls – Patty, Sue, Lil, June and Sandra. Neighbors. Friends. Loving parents. Good solid West Virginia stock.
- Robin Leone. Believer in good in all. Smart. Supporter of deeds. Giant in category of big hearts.
- Dr. William Phillips De Veaux, Elliott Bryant and Virgil Hodges. God's leaders and followers. Supporters of man's faith. Leaders in the value of education and of the heart.
- Dr. Nick Natiello. Wonderful friend. Commencement speaker. Respected in community leadership and business success around the world. Friend of many. Best friend of Naomi.
- Pastor John Crosby. A leader of congregations. A teacher of His teachings. A wonderful friend and example of good.

Acknowledgements

- Ray and Sheri Mehl. Superb examples of the medical and educational professions. Super friends and great parents.
- Jeff and Shari Mangas. He was there for me and she was an angel during my horrific riding horse accident. They are always there for others. Fine parents, good horse trainers and an excellent guide for financial issues.
- Gary Geiken represents the creed of the Boy Scouts of America. He is and lives that creed and what it stands for.
- Alex Plechash and Denise Kozejed. God's servants. Doing His work and sharing His glory.
- Tim and Lynn Fecteau are both a joy in our lives. They are artists, entertainers, chefs, sailors, and just wonderful family and friends.
- Tom and Valerie Gonser at www.gonzit.com are best examples of helping, giving and making introductions. Their faith is strong, family ties are unmovable, and their strength in making a difference in the lives of others is off the scale.
- Dan Dauffenbach, Scott and Jennifer Bremer and Deon and Kathy Kissoon. Representatives of all our wonderful Prior Lake and Minnesota neighbors. Everyone is always there for us. We are so blessed.
- Birgitta Rice. Always helping others especially in the field of diabetes. She is Mother Teresa in today's world.
- Bill and Carol Farb. Parents of Jason and nurturers of a wonderful gift to our family. We thank you.
- Bob and Joyce Lester. Best friends. Spiritual. Outstanding teacher and provider of gifts for teaching in China. Superb golfer and parents. Loving family and outstanding attorney.
- Pat Riggs. Financial genius. Eternal optimist. Dedicated father. Strong faith and filled with dignity. World traveler. His wife Cheryl is his best friend.

- Perry Williams. Great support and friend. Extraordinary promoter. A giant in helping others. The best.
- Theresa and Frank Gustafson. God's messenger for good. Supporters of children. Biggest hearts in the world. They challenge all of us to do better and be better. Recipients of their angel's wings early. Loving parents and best friends to many.
- Bob Haley. A masterful sales person within the technology arena. Always giving. True friend to many.
- Don Giacchetti. A blue ribbon winner of any racquetball court. Always wanting to help others. Giving, giving, giving. He's earned his stripes in life.
- Jacques Gibbs. The maestro of presentations. A friend and confidant to many. Always there. A teacher of life. A valued advisor for life's financial and personal challenges.
- Dr. David Osgood, MD. Left handed slugger. First base extraordinaire. Red Sox spokesperson. Friend not forgotten. Long time shadow in Green Fields.

Indulge me a moment longer. There are so many friends to thank for their support and for being in my life, including: Jay Abdo, Joseph Acri, Rich and Judy Adamkiewicz, Dr. Jan Thatcher Adams, Randy Adamsick, Cheryl Alexander, John Anderson, Kathy A. Anderson, Tamishia Anderson, Bev Asher, Dean Bachelor, Richard Barbacane, Robert Barnet, Michael Barrett, Tom Barry, Dee Bartolo, Bob Battle, Walter Battle, Guy Beach, Matthew Beck, Dale N. Beckmann, Cynthia Beiler, Brady Benson, Doug Benson, Jackie Berhardt, Fred and Anita Betterelli, Scott Blackburn, Angie Blackburn, Bob Blank, Jack Blesi, Marvin Block, Sara Blomberg, Jon Bolen, Kelsey Bourdeaux, Jim and Kris Bowers, Sherry Bowers, Dianne Boyer, Karen and Darrell Bramer, Brian Brantley, Tom Bregmann, Joe Brennen, Dan Brewer, James Brinegar, Tracy Brock, James D. Brown, Alice Bruno, Alexis Bryson,

Appendix

Rafael Bryson, Kenneth Budny, Stan Cahill, Arne H. Carlson, Pam Carlson, Steve Carlton, Bob Casey, Tom Cecchini, Bill Chambers, Serenity and Chris Charlebois, Rick Chiero, Brad Childs, Marlene Claire, Sara Classen, Ed and Lynn Cochrane, Buddy Cohen, Antoine Collins, Karl Collins, Tomica Collins, Mary Conant, Don Conlen, Beverly Connolly, Connie Connor, Felicia Cooper, Marcia Cooper, Ken Couri, Stephanie and Otis Courtney, Monica Cuevas, George Danko, John Dasburg, Stuart Dankers, Shirley Davis, Bill and Ginny Deinhammer, Brad Dennis, Roland Denton, Karleen Denton, Duane Derksen, Selena Dieringer, Greg Dittrich, Bob Dohaney, Maisey Doheny, Auriel Doheny, Leonard Donaldson, Dr. Chistina Donnell, Bill Drake, Ed Driscoll, Bill Duggan, Lynn Duprey, Marlene Earll, Al Edeker, Marian Wright Edelman, Richard Eichhorn, Jim and Polly Ekern, Bob Elzer, Gail Emerson, John and Kathy Engel, Dr. Donald Ericksen, Tom Erickson, Larry Ernster, Tom Esh, Joe Evan, Sara Fabie, Jason Farb, Lil Farrer, George and Judy Fead, Tim Fecteau, Lynn Fecteau, Frank Fecteau, Mollie Fecteau, Lil Fidler, Sandra Fidler, Mario Fernandez, J. Marie Fieger, Bob Fletcher, Mary Ellen Foley, Glenn Ford, Judye Foy, Beverly Freeman, Stasa Fritza, Chester Gadzinski, Tom Gegax, Brian Gaggan, Walter Gansser, Kyle and Michelle Gearhart, Gary Geiken, June Gendron, Raymond Gendron, Carl George, Wilson Gewarges, Don Giacchetti, Jake Gibbs, Tom and Val Gonser, Sandy and Tom Gratny, Keith and Connie Greiman, Roderick Griggs, Ernie Griffes, Troy Gronseth, Allan Grosh, Kent Grosser, Karl Gruhn, Arlie Gunderman, Dave Gundersen, Tina M. Haapala, Rod Haenke, Bob Haley, David and Lucille Hamelin, Susan and Doug Hamley, Neal Hardek, Alice Hardy, Charles Hardy Jr., Debbie Hardy, Clarissa Hardy, Felicia Hardy, Alice Hardy, Terry Harris, Pam Harris, Ashley Hart, Karen Hatchett, Rick Hauser, Peter Ludwig Hauser, Wes Hayne, Merrie Healy, Robert Hegland, Steve Heim, Greg Heinemann, Marie Hidem, Jenny Higgins, Richard Hocks, Kathy Hoekstra, Gerald Hoffman, Gregg Hoffman, Pat Hoffman, Robert Hoffman, Gary Holland, Natalie Homa, Wendy Homa, Thomas J. Horak, Dock Houk,

Bill Howe, Elise Howe, Marilyn and Earl Hubbard, Donna Rice Hughes, Carey Humphries, Deborah Jackson, Ralph Jacobson, Tom Jacoby, Kelly K. Jahner-Byrne, Ken Janusz, Jerry Jenko, Ruby Jerus, Timothy Jett, Ted Jewitt, Nancy Joffre, Pat Johnson, Candy Johnson, Walter Josten, Marty Kanter, Harvie Kasina, Jack Kelly, Mike Kelly, Willie Kelly, William Kerney, Nelli Kim, Carolyn Ann Kink, Barry Kinsey, Larry Kline, Brad Klukas, Faith Knight, Jim Kretsch, David Kronemeyer, Jean Kronemeyer, Tom Krupp, Barb Krupp, Betsy Krupp, Dennis Kuchenmeister, Charles Kuivinen, Vito Kuraitis, Robin Kutz, Lily Lai, John Lamb, Kelly Langdon, Norm and Joyce Lanpher, Reginald Larcholey, Gene Larkin, Karen and Ted Larkin, Kent Larson, Dan Lawrence, Suzanne Leavitt, Ben LeComte, Tony Lee, Rae Ann Lenway, Dr. Arthur Leon, Gary Lesley, Bob Lester, Joyce Lester, John Lipps, Joan Lowe, Lonnie L. Lowe, Shirley F. Lowe, Patricia Lowe, Mark Lynch, Jim Lynn, Doug Lyons, Carole Mackew, Brad Madson, Ed Mall, Jeff Mangas, Sherry Mangas, Zak Manuszak, Nina Marklund, Doug Marshall, Forler Massnick, Carrie Massnick, John Mattson, Joyce Morse-Mayhew, John McGuire, Robert McLean, David McNally, Estelle McWilliams, David McWilliams, Alexander McWilliams Jr., Gary McWilliams, Kevin McWilliams, Molly Mehl, Ron Mehl, Ray Mehl, Sharon Mehl, Chris Meyer, Dan and Carol McGowen, William Mikial, Dan Miller, Dave Miller, Judy Miller, Terry Millinger, Fred Montana, Joe Monteith, David Monteith, David and Ellen Mooney, Terry Moore, John Moore, Dorothy Moore, John Morris, Mike Morris, Carol Mott, Nancy Murphy, Lisa Myers, Bruce Myers, Rick Myre, Nick Natiello, Rick Nelles, Kevin Nelson, Monique Nelson, Richard Newman, Anne Nicolai, Sonya Nolan, Don Norris, David Nye, Emily O'Dell, Hazel O'Leary, Patrice L. Olive, David Olson, David Osgood, Erin Ostler, Robert Ostrow, Jessie Overton, Eric Paczosa, James Pagliarini, Chuck Parten, Tom Payne, Bill Pearson, Bill Peck, Carol Peck, Edna Peck, Donald Peck, Tom Peck, Ryan Peck, Connor Peck, Stacy Peck, Jim and Cindy Perry, Joshua Scott Perry, James J. Pesis, David Peterson, Reid Peterson, Tom Petters, Michael

Acknowledgements

W. Phillips, Norm Picard, Julia Pointer, Alex Plechash and Denise Kozojed, John and Marlene Pope, Joseph Porter, Shirley F. Porter, Larry Potter, Douglas Phillip Powell, Paul Price, Leonard Przybylski, Jan Radke, Rick Rainbolt, David Rasmussen, Dr. Tim Ratorja, Chuck Rauenhorst, Christopher Reese, Kit Reynolds, Jerry Rice, Pat and Cheryl Riggs, Jovelyn Richards, Phillip Roche, Brian Rocqmore, Mae Rodgers, Sara Rogers, Mike Rommel, Wil Rose, Kathy Roseberry, David Ross, Lynn Rudisill Warner, Bill Rudkin, Beverly Ruse, George W. Ryan, Richard Saliterman, Steve Salmen, John Salstrom, Rick Sandlin, Ron Sanders, Terry Sandvold, John Schmaedeke, Kathy Schmidt, Dick Schultz, Glenn Seefeldt, Dan Seeman, Ed Sewell, Marshall Seybold, Fortina Seybold, Steve Shamblot, Stephen Shank, Don Shelby, Kevin Sheridan, Sue Shimalla, Thomas M. Shivetts, Scott Shragg, Julie Shogren and Shane Krey, Stuart Shwiff, Pam Silverman, Nancy Simms, Caroline Sloth, Mary Smith, Paul Robert Smith, Shirley Smith, Tom and Nancy Solem, Dr. Brent Sorenson, Annette Spears, Lynnise Spears, Dave St. Peter, Erika Stacey, Durward Starr, John Stearns, Bill Steele, Clifford Steele, Joan Steffend, Michelle Steinhoff, Helen Strusacker, Mark Stump, Jim Sullivan, Dr. Alan Serposs, Doralee Suther, James Sutter, Glenn Swann, Jolea Swann, Sandy Hill Sweetser, Sal Tarraf, Jane Tarraf, Jim Taylor, Beth Terrell, Bob Terry, Tony Thomas, Brad Thompson, David Thompson, Jay Thompson, Katie Thompson, Sandi Thompson and Norm Nominee, Tom Toole, Charlie Thorpe, Jeff Turner, Violette Turner, Bob Twiss, Fred Ulrich, Avery Van Goard, Cathy Van Maren, Ellen Velasco-Thompson, Tim VandeSteeg, Sarah Verduzco, Connie Vernon, Jeffrey Vest, Michael Vincent, Doug Vukson-Van Beek, Dawn Vukson-Van Beek, Iris Waade, Robbie Waade, Robert Waade, Brett Waldman, Mark Walk, Brack Ward, John Warder, Dr. Charles O. Watkin, Gordon Watson, Julie Weier, Bud WeiserSenator Paul Wellstone, Shirlee Wendroth, Mary Wescott, Don and Gailee Westlund, Deb Weston, Jude and Shirley Weyrauch, Mike Wheelock, Mitch White, Aleane White, Terry White, Lorene Whitson, Stewart Widdess, John Williams, Tim Wilson,

Timothy M. Wilson, David Wolfe, Perry Williams, Tom Wolfgram. John Yonker, Eric Young, Dick and Marie Yutendale and Gerald Zeno.

Thank you, sincerely, to all my heroes shown here and also those found throughout this book in each picture and each word – and to those I may have misplaced.

Terry Hitchcock

P.S. Today, I am blessed with my life, my family, Mary Ann my best friend, and the friends who surround me each day with their support and love. My faith is strong and although I have no intention of running marathons again, I continue to explore how I might give back, make differences in the lives of others, and to believe as well as teach others that the difficult things we do immediately, and the impossible we take a little more time.

Acknowledgements

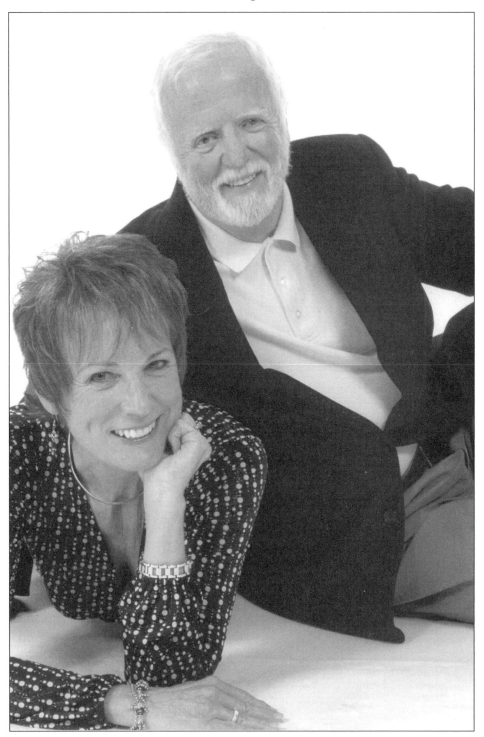

A Fathers Odyssey

THE AUTHORS

TERRANCE S. HITCHCOCK

Born in Vermont. Air Force Veteran. Married to Mary Ann. Blended five children. Currently living in Prior Lake, Minnesota. His previous book was "American Business: The Last Hurrah?" Written numerous articles on business subjects. Teaches "Leadership and Ethics" at Metropolitan State University. Entrepreneur and public speaker on life issues. Doctorate in business, a law degree and honorary degrees.

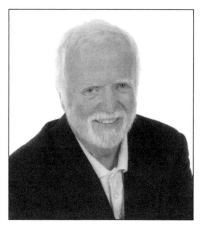

PETER JESSEN

Raised in the Northwest. Currently lives in Portland, Oregon. MA in Sociology and doctoral studies at Rutgers University. Vietnam Era Veteran. Infantry Officer Candidate School. Consultant to three national commissions, the Smithsonian Institution, and hundreds of individual executives. Headed communication consulting firms in McLean Virginia and New York City. Co-author of "The Minneapolis Story Through My Eyes"

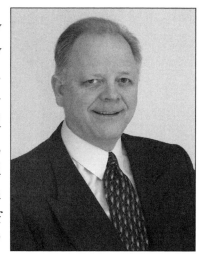

BEHIND THE SCENES

KYLE GEARHART

Kyle Gearhart is an award-winning journalist, an entrepreneur and a consultant. He is the proud father of two children, and enjoys traveling with his wife. He is an avid runner who enjoys the ease of a 5K and the pace of a 10K. Armed with a master's of journalism degree and a master's of business degree, Kyle dreams of building a media empire that both serves and challenges its readers.

JEFFREY TURNER

Jeffrey Turner is the author of two novels and four novellas, and has written screenplays for numerous independent film companies. He is a long-time guest at the AggieCon science fiction and fantasy convention, and teaches an annual writing workshop there. Although not a runner himself, Jeff enjoys hiking and traveling the world, and is the happy father of two wonderful girls. In addition to writing he works as a business analyst for Microsoft, and lives in Fort Worth with his wife and daughters

TIM VANDESTEEG

Over the past decade Mr. VandeSteeg has directed, produced and written independent feature films, commercials, and promotional television shows (EPKs, PSAs, interstitials, and behind-the-scenes pieces) for such high-profile clients as ABC, SUBWAY, and Hallmark Entertainment. Mr. VandeSteeg has been featured in such national newspapers, magazines and books as; "The New York Times", "Daily Variety", "Hollywood Reporter", "TNT Roughcuts", "Minneapolis Star and Tribune" and "The Writer's Guide to Hollywood". Mr. VandeSteeg is the CEO of Indiewood Pictures (www.

indiewoodpictures.net), an independent film development and production company. Recently, Mr. VandeSteeg directed, produced, and co-wrote the award-winning love story "Fall Into Me", and is currently producing and directing the new documentary; "My Run" and in development of the inspirational motion picture "Pushing Life", both based on the life story of Terry Hitchcock. www.myrunmovie.com.

KAREN LARKIN

Superb, superb…and then some. Creative professional with computer graphics.

BRAD LEE THOMPSON

Creative designer and producer of educational programs and successful author of more than a dozen books.

AN APPROACH TO LIVING
LIFE'S DAILY MARATHONS

It is my pleasure to introduce to you some of the wisdom of my friend Peter Jessen. Peter is a seminar and workshop motivational trainer and speaker. We have worked together off and on since the 1990s in various consulting and training contexts. His friendship and guidance in structuring lists to achieve goals was one of the reasons I was able to complete my two thousand-mile journey to Atlanta in 1996. My thanks to him.

ORGANIZATIONAL HABITS

Written by Peter Jessen

One of the questions everyone should consider is, "what is your GPA, or goals per action?" In other words, do your actions and your daily steps serve your goals? If the answer is *no*, then you need to reassess your actions and how you allocate your time. Why do we need to do so? In the book *The Social Construction of Reality*, sociologist Peter Berger clues us into the importance of developing roles and the routines that sustain them. In *Facilitating Treatment Adherence*, the cognitive-behavioral psychologist Donald Meichenbaum and his colleague Dennis Turk, a professor of psychiatry, demonstrate empirically that the simple key to making goals is to make lists. Thus, list the routines and scripts for your different roles.

Think of the lists you create as road maps to your goals, just as Terry needed road maps for his Run. Terry had to take steps forward, to make strides, and turn the map into reality. So do you. Terry had to develop a new role for himself, the role of runner, and he had to develop routines to maintain that role, routines dealing with daily exercise, sleep, and diet. So do you. Using another metaphor, think of these lists as recipes to follow, to bake whatever cakes of life you have in mind. The key to developing the best ingredients that work is to define your roles and then develop routines to practice daily.

Lists help you set goals and evaluate how well you are doing in meeting your goals. To make it easier, break your goals down into objectives, then break these objectives down into procedures with time targets. These are the ingredients for your to-do lists. List the time schedule, the resources, and the people you need to reach your goals. Then commit to your lists, as Terry committed to his Run. Review your lists every day and make a new one for the following day. At the end of each month review your lists for positive patterns to refine and patterns you want to change or eliminate. Use this month-end review to redefine your roles and routines to meet your goals.

Customize your own list of affirmations to include positive things about you now and the positive things you would like to see about yourself in the future. Thus, define your roles and routines and affirm them. Use these then to customize a list of affirmation principles to guide your personal and professional roles and routines (behavior). The affirmation principles become motivational statements to repeat. Recite the list in the morning and at night before bed. What you recite so will you become. So be careful. You are putting together a powerful list. It will enable you to take the steps necessary to run your daily marathons, to make your dreams and goals come true.

Incorporate the lists and goals into your daily organizational habits to facilitate becoming a more effective person in your roles as mentor and teacher at home, at work, and in your community, neighborhood, church and school.

One of life's difficulties is remaining inspired and motivated. One of the best ways to do this is through the greatest influences in our lives: the people we associate with and the books we read. Charlie "Tremendous" Jones, a motivational speaker and author, said "You're the same person today you will be five years from now except for two things: the people you meet and the books you read." When it comes to friends and associates, choose wisely. When it comes to books, you should read those that grab your fancy.

QUOTES

"Terry's life's story is an incredible inspiration of how anyone with a dream can achieve so much by just never ever giving up! Even more remarkable is how Terry has been able to touch the lives of so many families and inspire our nation's youth who are our leaders of tomorrow. This is a must have book for every family's library!"
 —*Dave Anderson, founder of Famous Dave's restaurants.*

"Life is challenging and rarely fair – Terry's own life is a testament to that fact. His own story of dedication, determination and overcoming is inspiring for many generations to come. Thank you Terry for being such a wonderful example of God's love by reaching out to show all parents they can make a difference by accepting responsibility instead of blaming or making excuses. The world owes us nothing – we owe the world – to be the best we can possibly be. Terry, you are a World Changer!"
 —*Tom and Valerie Gonser, creators of www.gonzit.com.*

"When I think of life from near its end I am increasingly conscious of legacy. Like the relay team member I am more conscious of how well I pass the baton, not whether I won... Terry Hitchcock is my life example. He calls it driven. I call it passion. The result is the same. Lives changed, turned around, and a lot more "can do" people out there than before Terry came into their lives with a walk and talk that is convincing."
 —*David Durenberger, a U.S. Senator for Minnesota from 1978 to 1995, now serving as Senior Health Policy Fellow at the University of St. Thomas in Minneapolis, Minn.*

"As a Minnesota Senator and Attorney, I have always felt privileged to be able to help and guide others – to be a beacon of hope for many. We all should share in that passion. True everyday heroes such as Terry and his son Chris are examples of individuals who challenge all of us to step up and make a difference in the lives of many. Let us all remember our obligations to be there for others."
 —*U.S. Sen. Michele M. Bachmann, of Minnesota.*

"Terry is one of the most driven and dedicated people that I have met. Running from Minneapolis to Atlanta is an amazing example of setting a goal and doing whatever it takes to reach it. One of the motivators that Terry uses is the one thing that impresses me the most: he is always thinking of other people, especially children, and what he can do that would benefit them. He has an innate gift of being able to touch the lives of others, and he uses it to his fullest potential."
—*Scott Meier, a physical education teacher and strength & conditioning coach in Farmington Public Schools in Minnesota. He trained Terry for his Run.*

"When Terry Hitchcock gave his motivational speech to my summer camp for inner city kids, I told them Terry's message was right on target, one of the best I had ever heard, and if they really wanted to succeed in life, they would follow what Terry said. The same thing goes for the players on my team and anyone else wanting to achieve personal and professional success."
—*Dennis Green, former head coach of the Minnesota Vikings and the Arizona Cardinals and a driving force behind many youth and community development programs.*

"Heroes come in all shapes and sizes. But to me, the real heroes, on and off the ball field, are the men and women who overcome adversity to stay with their families and raise their children. Terry Hitchcock ran the "MegaMarathon '96" to draw attention to the help needed by kids, especially kids in single parent households. Terry's message is an inspiration to all who read his story."
—*Gene Larkin, former Minnesota Twins who batted in the winning run of the 1991 World Series.*

"I find Terry's story and his mountain-moving faith definitely worth listening to. Being a paraplegic (due to a construction accident 25 years ago), I have had my own challenges, and I often need to hear the journey of others like Terry to keep my own faith alive and know that my own Grand Canyon dreams can become a reality if God is in them."
—*Bob Bardwell, a motivational speaker and inspirational leader, founder and director of Ironwood Springs Christian Ranch, and a winner of three Twin Cities Marathons and a 1988 top ten National Marathon racer.*

"I was so moved by Terry's story that I have included it in my new book of essays on ordinary men and women who have become extraordinary heroes for our time."
—*Rudy Ruettiger, a motivational speaker and the inspiration for the film "Rudy".*

"In essence, Terry and his son, Chris, successfully completed their own quest. His 2,000 miles was a Feat of Feet. He experienced endurance at the highest of levels. He challenged the impossible – and won. He did it for all the right reasons – our kids and their families."

—Dan Beuttner, an explorer and educator who has bicycled across five continents and set three Guinness World Records.

"Terry Hitchcock and his son, Chris, have inspired us with their commitment to kids and families... Their remarkable 2,000-mile journey to Atlanta serves as a truly powerful reminder to us all: We must take advantage of opportunities in our own lives to help each other in our own daily marathons."

—U.S. Rep. Jim Ramstad of Minnesota, first elected to Congress in 1990, a member of the House Ways and Means Committee and the Health and Trade Subcommittees.

"Knowing Terry as his doctor, I will never cease to be amazed at what he has done, persevering through all that pain and loneliness, plus a heart attack. He has shown us all the power of the heart. When a dream and a vision come from the depths of one's heart, anything can be accomplished – defying all barriers! I am grateful for what he has done to inspire me and all of humanity to transcend our limits. Therein lays our Godliness."

—Meghabhuti Roth, M.D., a family medical practitioner, friend, and avid marathon runner.

"The success of Men's Wearhouse over the last quarter century has been built by ordinary people doing extraordinary things. We all have the potential within us, and every day provides opportunities to decide to become extraordinary – just like Terry Hitchcock did on his inspirational 2,000-mile journey. I guarantee it!"

—George Zimmer, co-founder and CEO of the Men's Wearhouse.

"A story that needs to be told over and over again. Everyone needs to support and share Terry's vision that children are our future. We all need to help."

—William H. Philipp, Jr., vice president, Lifelong Learning, Adult Learning Service PBS.

"One of the great problems of adults is that they either don't or can't dream. They need models for how to do so. Terry provides that in his book. Every adult will be a step closer to achieving their dreams after they read Terry's book."

—Ron Saunders, president of business sales at Sprint.

"Terry has found a way to help others, one by one, as he encountered them on his Run and as he encounters them, one on one, as they read his book. When people like Terry help people help themselves; they make it easier for us."
—*Pam Carlson, director of advertising and promotion for United Way*

"Terry Hitchcock is a man with a mission, an exemplar role model who is devoted to children and their welfare, as well as adding new meaning to their lives."
—*Jonathan Waterman, adventurer and author of "Arctic Crossing: 2,000 Miles Across the Northeast Passage" and eight other books.*

"In the entertainment business, greatness is exemplified by playing on the edge, discovering the delicate balance between innovation and absolute strength. Terry runs in that same pack. He exemplifies believing in a dream, and implementing the dream, the faith where one man can make the difference."
—*LaSalle Gabriel, Grammy award-winning guitarist, music producer and president and chief executive officer of LGI Entertainment.*

"The choices we make determine not only our character but also the quality of our life. Terry Hitchcock and his kids – Chris, Jason and Teri Sue – believed enough in each other to support their dad's dream and to totally believe that he would succeed. To many, it seemed an impossible dream. To Terry's kids, nothing is impossible if you believe in yourself."
—*Sandra Humphrey, author of "If you had to choose, what would you do?", "Keepin It Real", and other books.*

"Most of my life has been spent in and around the realm of stories. The ones that always unlock my soul are the stories of triumphant struggle, ceaseless determination and undying spiritual faith. Terry Hitchcock's life story of faith in action is one of those stories that will touch anyone who hears it."
—*Craig Rice, motion picture artist, entertainment company executive and educator.*

"These days, inspirational is a much overused adjective, and often a sales pitch is attached. With Terry, the inspiration is always genuine and carries no price tag except to experience."
—*Frank Kinikin, head of film and television development, Stellar Sports and Entertainment, Seoul, Korea.*

"Terry Hitchcock's story is an inspiration for anyone interested in the future of our children. Terry's life is a testament to persistence, faith and sacrifice."
—*Ann Tatlock, author and the winner of the Silver Angel Award.*

"Terry's life story and the work he does on behalf of others are inspirational. His determination to live, love and give in the face of overwhelming challenges is an example that is needed in our culture today. Terry's commitment to the welfare of children is a testament to the power of love and selfless giving."
    —*CH (MAJ) John Morris, Minnesota Army National Guard, Chaplain for returning veterans from the war.*

"The future of this country is its children. We should honor our kids and we should honor their parents just as Chris and Terry did. Our kids, our parents, our families – these are the real everyday heroes."
    —*Dr. Nick Natiello, business consultant, and executive.*

"Last year my brother Michael and I started to realize that a lot of kids are poor. They don't have enough food to eat. They don't have many toys or clothes. And they don't have a place to put their stuff. To help these people, we started collecting backpacks and supplies. I know this is something that God wants us to do. He wants us to help people."
    —*Robbie Chance, age 8, Shakopee, Minnesota. Co-founded the Everybody Needs a Backpack program in 2002.*

"Every kid needs somebody to help and love them. They might not know who we are, but that's OK. We should help and love them anyway."
    —*Michael Chance, age 6, Shakopee, Minnesota. Co-founded the Everybody Needs a Backpack program in 2002.*

"In today's world, our kids and families are faced with significant challenges and obstacles to achieving their dreams. Even so, we should never give up on our dreams. Dreams do come true. We should always believe."
    —*Lt. Colonel Ernest J. Griffes, Base Commander of the General Patton Army Air Field in Chiriaco Summit, California.*

"Terry Hitchcock beat the odds, courageously forged through barriers and ultimately achieved the impossible. He joins the many men and women who founded this country and continue to keep this country remembering that freedom from bondage, yokes of tyranny, and oppression are nasty taskmasters. Whether these taskmasters are self imposed or imposed by tyrants, they must be removed and replaced with strength, power and authority."
    —*Dr. LuAnn Walters, voice of Talk Education Radio and founder of the One Room Schools Foundation.*

"I met Terry as a consultant to his organization, the Heroes and Dreams Foundation. … As you learn more about Terry and his own limitations, it is easy to see his message; no matter how difficult things look, you can overcome any obstacles."
   —*John Bianchi, Principal*

"I admire Terry as a person."
   —*Don Stolz, Founder, Old Log Theater*

"Only worry about the things that you can control and you should always have complete control of your attitude. You have two choices – positive or negative. Show a kid a positive attitude and a smile, and they will show you the zest for life that will make you feel like a kid again.… Heroes give something much more valuable than money. They give their time and their heart. Keep running Terry!"
   —*Joe Schmit, president of the media and marketing group for Petters Group Worldwide and previously news and sports anchor for Channel 5 Eyewitness News / KSTP TV in Minneapolis.*

"We come alone, we leave alone. And in between, we sing alone… So dance we must and thrash our swords… And run not from but at and towards." You fit that, Terry. And I think you can well relate to that. I appreciate what you are trying to achieve and it is certainly noble and worthy and full of virtue. Lord knows we are in dire need of just that thing. Real Heroes help make dreams real for real people, especially the kids. That makes you a Hero in my book. Good luck and Godspeed and see you at the Finish!"
   —*Gary Lesley, president of Head Lites Corp., St. Paul, Minn.*

"Each of us is called to make a difference in the world. I hope that Terry's story helps others to hear their own calling and respond."
   —*Gregory R. Palen, on the board of directors of numerous corporations, including Polaris Industries and Valspar.*

"One of the great problems of adults is that they either don't dream or can't dream. They need role models for how to do so. Terry provides that in his book. Every adult will be a step closer to achieving their dreams after they read Terry's book."
   —*Ron Saunders, president of business sales for Sprint/Nextel.*

"Terry is a real-life role-model for all those who need proof that the negotiation of obstacles and adversity can provide powerful building blocks for a life of contribution and service. Bouncing back again and again from astounding challenges, he sends a powerful beacon into the future which lights the way for the children of the world. Hope, Service, and Family are the electricity powering his remarkable vision and accomplishment. He is the living example of his ideas about Everyday Heroes."
—*Jan Thatcher Adams, M.D.*

"Champions focus on where they are going verses what they have been through. Terry and Chris are the ultimate examples. They are driven by passion and guided by a deep, authentic desire to make a difference in the lives of our youth. In my opinion, Terry and Chris are American heroes!"
—*Ricky Rainbolt, founder of Rainbolt's Thundering Seminars.*

"Each of us has our own marathons to run. Terry and Chris ran for us and showed us the way. Our families and our kids, all need our support. They have their dreams as we have ours. Let's all run our marathons together and see our dreams come true. Two thousand miles isn't that far, is it?"
—*Robert Hegland, businessman.*

"Greatness is something that all athletes strive for. What Terry has accomplished I will always think of as an amazing accomplishment. He is truly someone who inspires me as an athlete."
—*Lindsay Whalen, WNBA point guard with the Connecticut Suns.*

"This book proves that a single step is not only gigantic but affirms the very fact that we are alive! Well done, Terry."
—*Jim MacLaren, founder of the Choose Living Foundation and an actor, writer, motivational speaker, retired professional athlete and quadriplegic.*

"Being defeated is temporary. Giving up makes it permanent."

—*Dan and Jeri Blomberg represent an example for all of us to follow, of the love and faith that a couple can have in their role as parents and as partners in life. Jeri, although dealing herself with Raynaud's syndrome and Scleroderma, partners with Dan to provide a home full of love and gentle support. Their four children – Daniel IV, Michael, Sarah and Alysia are the special gifts that God has given them. Their love and dedication to their family literally overflows, each day helping Michael, who is profoundly disabled with Autism, Seizure disorder and mental retardation and Alysia, who has Cerebral Palsy, Cortical blindness, Seizure disorder and is microcephalic. Both children live at home, are very happy, and loved and cherished by their other brother and sister, Daniel and Sarah, who live in other parts of the country and who visit their parents and brother and sister as much as possible. A remarkable family, filled with love, and an example of true family togetherness. An example for all to follow.*

"Much which passes as revealed wisdom in my realm, if truth be told, came from my father. While he gave me much thoughtful advice, it was a simple story he shared with me, not to instruct or inspire – but to share a piece of his life, that has formed my own.

"He told me that when he was a young adult, he got into a very rare argument with his mother whom he loved with all his heart. He said some cross words and stormed from the house. While he was gone, his mother passed away. She had suffered for years with a bad heart, and it gave out. Nothing he had said or she had done had brought it on.

"What hurt my father the most was that the last words his mother heard from him were not the words of love he felt in his heart. He vowed, from that day forward, to treat everyone he met as though it would be the last time he ever saw them. As important, he behaved as though it would be the last time anyone ever saw him."

—*Don Shelby, WCCO-TV anchor and reporter and winner of three Emmy's and two Peabody Awards.*

"When life hands you a negative, don't despair; it just might turn into a great picture."

—*Michael Vincent, singer and songwriter.*

"Goals in a lifetime are merely dreams without action. Our Children deserve parents and mentors who will take action on their behalf to inspire and motivate them to change the world in a positive way like Terry."

—*Gregory D. Dittrich, attorney.*

"The two main responsibilities of life are personal development and service to others. No one is more important than children. Not only planning directs us, but inspiration as well. … Where does the inspiration and tenacity that Terry demonstrated come from? Where does one's public service toward the common good come from, especially for children and the less fortunate? For me, it comes from the still small voice of God, heard from people, orally, reading or just experiencing their presence."
—*Albert H. Quie, former Minnesota governor, state senator and member of the U.S. Congress.*

"I have known Terry for over 25 years as his former neighbor, colleague, business partner and friend and I can tell you that his dedication to and love of kids of all ages and their dreams has never wavered or ceased to amaze me. Terry was called to make a difference in this world and even though he has faced untold challenges he always believed in himself, overcame adversity and never gave up – becoming a positive role model and forging new footprints for us all to follow. His vision, passion, desires and dreams for kids are unheard of and I am happy that this book will finally tell his long overdue story for all to hear."
—*David Mooney, President & CEO, Boundless Expectations LLC, Los Angeles CA, www.boundlessexpectations.com*

"Each day, we have opportunities that are given us to share, develop and to support others. God blesses us each moment and we need to be aware of what He challenges us to do. Terry and Chris were blessed to be able to travel their 2,000 miles in a trek that was called impossible. They were able to accomplish their dream because they believed. Each one of us needs to see God's gifts and to appreciate His blessings."
—*Chuck Kuivenen, department head of the School of Business at Northwestern College.*

"One of my all time favorite quotes is Martin Luther King Jr's "I have a dream …". No matter what you dream nor how high you aim, you can be sure of one thing, if you believe and work at it, your dreams will come true."
—*Colleen Needles Steward, founder and president of Tremendous! Entertainment, a television production and distribution company based in Minneapolis.*

"You can give a man a fish or teach him how to fish. We can give a kid life or we can teach him how to live. Any time we can spend enriching the lives of today's youth is time we are insuring a better quality life for tomorrow's youth."
    —*Bob Fisher, "Shoe" Bob has raised more than $5,500,000 for the Interfaith Outreach ministry.*

"Terry Hitchcock has always impressed me with his persistence and determination. He has much wisdom to share."
    —*David McNally, best selling author of "Even Eagles Need A Push".*

"I trained for and ran my first marathon at the age of 38 to cope with the tragic death of a 31-year-old staff member in the computer science department that I led at that time. My five-year-old daughter, Sasha, thought I was crazy. During her teenage years, running races together was just about the only activity Sasha wanted to do with me. Last fall Sasha, then 21, asked me to run with her in her first marathon with the goal of qualifying for Boston. We both qualified and ran Boston this year in the middle of a nor'easter. … When I think about Terry and his son Chris and the amazing challenge they took on together, I'm impressed not just by the unbelievable achievement of running 75 marathons in 75 days, but the vision and courage it took to set that goal. The world needs more people like Terry."
    —*Maria M. Klawe, president of Harvey Mudd College.*

"There are two attitudes that have served me well in my life, whether things seem to be going well at the moment or not. They are, no matter where you are, expect great things from life and yourself, and to be grateful for what is already there. It's a starting for hope and peace."
    —*Joan Steffend, host of HGTV's Decorating Cents and Emmy award winner.*

"Whether it's the game of golf or the game of life, we all need to do our part to nurture our children – our future – so that we all finish successfully on the 18th green. Terry and Chris did their par; they hit it straight and hit each green. We all can play. Let's tee off together. We can par each hole and once in awhile even make a birdie."
    —*Loyal H. "Bud" Chapman, artist and a golf amateur, in the truest sense of the word.*

"Kipling wrote in the classic poem, "IF": "If you can dream, but not make dreams your master; if you can think, and not make thoughts your aim; if you can meet with triumph and disaster and treat those two imposters just the same …

"Many of us have fond memories of fathers or grandfathers reading this entire poem to us as boys, often with personal examples attached. As we mature and acquire experiences of our own, we meet all the characters if Kipling's poem.

"It has been my privilege to work alongside Terry in several business settings, and in each he has exhibited extraordinary Constancy, perseverance, and strength of character. He has illustrated in his life what Kipling wrote with his pen."
—*Brad Childs, venture capitalist and real estate executive.*

"We all have the opportunity to be heroes everyday to someone, especially young people. The adventure in life is to discover, look for, recognize, and act on the ones that cross our paths in the normal course of events."
—*Mary Kiffmeyer, former Minnesota Secretary*

"We need always to be focused on the lives of our children everywhere and to make certain that they are not abandoned, but nourished, loved and respected. Terry's efforts contribute to those important steps."
—*Judy Miller, Executive Director of the Conrad N. Hilton Humanitarian Prize.*

"Terry is an amazing man. His drive and his will and dedication are contagious. We met a lot of wonderful people on the Children are Forever project. I really wanted to help to make a difference for single parents and their children. I know many friends and colleagues who are single parents and who need support and assistance. Finding quality childcare is hard. Terry's message is this: you can do anything you really want to do – even after a heart attack. You can do what you put your mind to. Because of Terry's story, I'm inspired that I too can do things and make a difference."
—*J. Marie Fieger is a member of the Minnesota Television and Film Board and President of Nemer Fieger Inc., a national public relations firm.*

"We need always to be focused on the lives of our children everywhere and to make certain that they are not abandoned, but nourished, loved and respected. Terry's efforts contribute to those important steps."
—*J. Marie Fieger is a member of the Minnesota Television and Film Board and President of Nemer Fieger Inc., a national public relations firm.*

"Terry is a real-life role model for all those who need proof that the negotiation of obstacles and adversity can provide powerful building blocks for a life of contribution and service. Bouncing back again and again from astounding challenges, he sends a powerful beacon into the future which lights the way for the children of the world. Hope, Service, and Family are the electricity powering his remarkable vision and accomplishment. He is the living example of his ideas about Everyday Heroes."
—*Jan Thatcher Adams, M.D.*

"Children are our most important resource. Providing them with safety, health and a supportive community is our greatest challenge. Thank you, Terry."
—*Julian Bond is Chairman of the Board of the NAACP, the oldest and largest civil rights organization in the United States. The holder of twenty-one honorary degrees, he is a Distinguished Professor at American University in Washington, DC, and a Professor in history at the University of Virginia.*

"Terry attempted the impossible – but he did it. He did it for kids. Everyone needs to know Terry's story. He is an icon for kids everywhere. Terry and his son, Chris, are heroes."
—*Tom Cecchini was an NFL Coach for the Minnesota Vikings and Collegiate Coach for the University of Iowa, Tulane University, Xavier University and the University of Michigan. He has received All-American and Big Ten honors.*

"Like Terry, I too have suffered the loss of a wife and was then graced with a second wife who has made my life worth living again. My life-long dream has been to play Al Jolson, ever since I heard him when I was ten. I accomplished my dream. Terry too is a dreamer. He is a living testament to the power of dreaming dreams and achieving them no matter what the obstacle."
—*Mike Burstyn starred in the national tour of The Allergist's Wife with Valerie Harper. Mike has also starred in the musical Jolson. Mike is an international entertainer on stage, screen and television, performing in nightclubs and concert stages throughout the world — in eight languages. His audiences have included Presidents, Queens and Prime Ministers. Mike has won two Israeli "Oscars" and was host of one of the most popular shows in The Netherlands, Belgium and Luxembourg.*

"Terry recognized that many people struggle along their path and stumble and fall and want to not get up and continue. Terry is a man who stood up and created new footprints to follow in case we walk our daily path alone. He encourages others to do the same so that no one will have to walk their path alone."
—*Krista Stenhaug. Writer, Artist and multiple times guest on Oprah Winfrey Television Show*

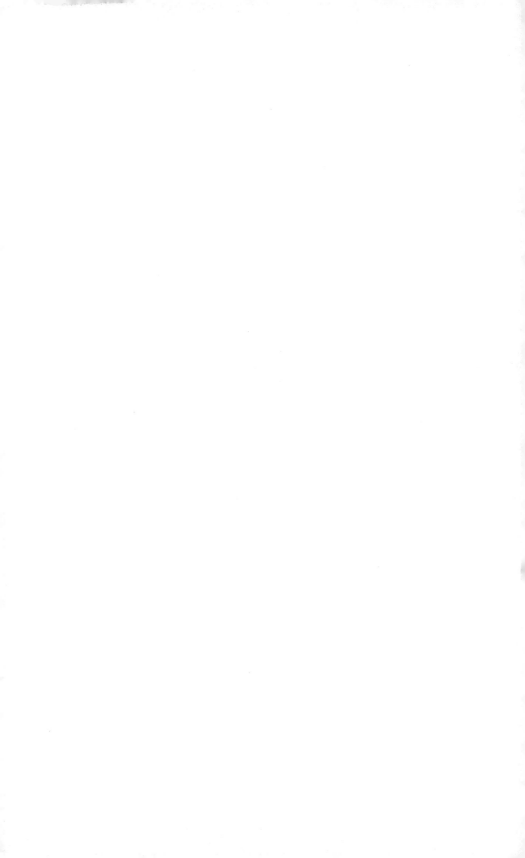